Portfolio development
and profiling for nurses
2nd edition

Central Health Studies

The Central Health Studies (CHS) series is designed to provide nurses and other health care professionals with up-to-date, informative texts on key professional and management issues and human skills in health care.

The Consulting Editor

The series was conceived by John Tingle,. B A Law Hons, Cert Ed, M Ed, Barrister, Senior Lecturer in Law, Nottingham Law School, Nottingham Trent University. John has published widely on the subject of the professional and legal accountability of health care professionals.

Other books in the series

Spiritual Care: A resource guide

Budgeting Skills: A guide for nurse managers

Patients' Rights, Responsibilities and the Nurse

Measuring the Effectiveness of Nurse Education: The use of performance indicators

Employment Law for Nurses

Research Appreciation: An initial guide for nurses and health care professionals

Management Skills for Community Nurses

Central Health Studies
Consulting Editor: John Tingle

Portfolio Development and Profiling for Nurses

Roswyn Brown

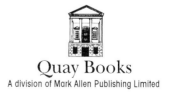

Quay Books
A division of Mark Allen Publishing Limited

Quay Books Division of Mark Allen Publishing Limited
Jesses Farm, Snow Hill, Dinton, Nr Salisbury, Wilts, SP3 5HN

©Mark Allen Publishing Ltd, 1995

British Library Cataloguing-in-Publication Data
A catalogue record for this book is available from the British Library

ISBN 1-85642-123-6

Printed in the UK by Butler & Tanner Limited, Frome & London

Contents

Chapter

Foreword   vii

Acknowledgements   ix

Preface   xi

1   Introducing portfolios and profiles   1

2   Creating your personal portfolio from your curriculum   13
     vitae

3   Enhancing the headings: from CV to portfolio   19

4   Goal setting and profiles for periodic registration   31

5   Profiles for continuing professional education   42

6   Putting your CATS among the profiles   61

7   An evaluation of a selection of profile packages   73

Appendix

1   Specimen curriculum vitae   81

2   UKCC PIN instructions   85

Glossary   87

Acronym list   91

Bibliography   93

Index   95

Foreword

It is with great pleasure that I welcome Roswyn Brown's second edition of her useful, practical guide to portfolios and profiles.

There is no doubt that the climate of change is creating a requirement for all nurses to be more aware of their past achievements and future needs. This has further been emphasised by the 'PREP & YOU' (1995) Information Pack distributed by the UKCC to each nurse earlier this year.

The articulation of professional nursing standards and the necessity to re-register every three years with the Council has led to an emphasis on nurses having the right kind of background, both professionally and educationally. This is clearly expressed in the UKCC's 'Future of Professional Practice' document from March 1994.

This book offers a clear, easy-to-follow route through the complexities of CVs, Portfolios and Profiles. Roswyn Brown has managed to avoid using the jargonistic language that raises barriers and limits the accessibility of knowledge and ideas. I would certainly recommend it to every nurse who is looking for a concise and helpful guide to what s/he should know about self-presentation for future opportunities (both in professional life and educationally).

Professor George Castledine

Acknowledgements

My first thanks must go to my family, Alan, Eleanor and Matthew, who have always supported me in the development of my own portfolio and profile. They have all contributed in very practical ways to the production of this book, not least by making the tea. Secondly, to a talented nurse tutor and colleague, Kath Butler, who patiently dealt with my bizarre ideas, masquerading as jokes and turned them into useful and amusing cartoons. She has, of course, placed the originals in her own personal portfolio.

My friend, Denise Robertson has been her usual ruthless self in pruning out the excess padding. Although I protested at the time, I am extremely grateful— a sentiment which I'm sure is shared by the reader.

I would also like to thank friends, colleagues and students who have been so generous in their support and criticism of the draft document.

Dedication

For my friend Valery Moran

......who always comes smiling through and to whom this second edition owes much.

Preface

Welcome to this second edition of Portfolio Development and Profiling for Nurses, which has been substantially updated with respect to current UKCC policy. The focus of the changes centres on the recent developments in relation to the interface between specialist and advanced practice.

The flexible and innovative approach that the Council is taking to these exciting developments means that opportunities for continuing education are still increasing at a phenomenal rate. The National Boards and the United Kingdom Central Council for Nursing, Midwifery and Health Visiting (UKCC) have played a crucial role in this, with initiatives which include Project 2000, PREP and the national frameworks for continuing education. Access to higher education is provided for increasing numbers of nurses at all stages of their careers, as the links between the profession and academic study develop and strengthen.

The choices confronting nurses may, at first, seem bewildering. These range from fulfilling the minimum statutory requirement (five days mandatory updating every three years) in order to remain in registered practice, to Masters' level work with advanced practitioner status. How far you progress between these two points will depend on you and your personal aspirations. However, whatever you choose to do, it is essential that you maintain a record of your professional and personal development. The main focus of this is to demonstrate what you have learned and how this contributes to your professional practice.

Personal professional portfolios or profiles can be used for a variety of purposes, and not just in relation to the statutory framework in which we practice. This short guide to Portfolio Development has deliberately adopted a more flexible approach, which offers you the choice to use your collection in a variety of ways for a variety of functions. This is why I have included discussions, not only on professional development, but also on your personal life experiences and achievements. We are, after all, being encouraged to develop 'unconventional careers' and to do this we must ensure that the gifts and talents that the whole person can bring to this are considered. I also believe that not to do so would strike at the very heart of what we are trying to achieve in terms of providing total client care. It is essential that we see and treat each other as unique individuals, acknowledging and taking into account the overlap between the private and public arenas of our lives. If we are not able to do this for ourselves, how can we possibly achieve it for the people we hope to serve?

The main reason for the production of portfolios is for the identification, development and release of talents and skills. These should be capable of responding to the changing health care needs of the population now, as well as promoting the development of new skills for the future. However, I have also been preoccupied over time by a concern about who cares for the carers; so this book is by way of a contribution towards that end, because portfolios should also provide the mechanism for mapping out satisfying life plans and optimising potential.

I hope this new edition will help you to get started on your own presentation, if you have not already done so, or give you some new ideas if you have. Here's to some happy reminiscing as you delve into the portmanteau of your past.

Good wishes for all those exciting developments in the future! Bon Voyage!

Roswyn Brown

> *Faculty of Health and Social Sciences*
> *University of Central England in Birmingham*

Chapter 1

Introducing Portfolios and Profiles

Introduction

Professor John Pilkington Hudson (1980) relates an amusing story of two schoolboys doing their homework. One said:

'We must be quiet because Granny is upstairs reading her bible.'

The other asked:

'Swotting for her finals?'

The variety of aspects that this book hopes to address currently concerns all nurses and may be seen in this schoolboy humour in terms of

1. the need to plan ahead according to your own individual needs and interests, both personally and professionally

2. the importance of continued development for both the novice nurse and the mature professional, particularly if you are to reach your potential

3. the value of due consideration and reflection on your past, current activities and future plans

To engage in these activities effectively, you are now expected to create and maintain a **personal portfolio or profile**.

What are personal portfolios and profiles?

The two terms are frequently used interchangeably in both the professional and higher education arenas. In their policy documents (1994, 1995), the United Kingdom Central Council (UKCC) refer to a **personal professional profile**, whereas the English National Board (ENB), as part of their development of the 'Framework for Continuing Professional Education' (1990), published a **Professional Portfolio** folder (1991).

For the purpose of this book, the term `**personal portfolio**' (which is an idea borrowed from graphic art and design) will be used in the following sense:

> '*A* **private** *collection of evidence which demonstrates the continuing acquisition of skills, knowledge, attitudes, understanding and achievement. It is both* **retrospective** *and* **prospective***, as well as reflecting the* **current** *stage of development and activity of the individual.*'

Such a definition conveys the notion that a **personal portfolio** can be all-embracing. It may include data from a variety of sources which are capable of conveying to others our qualities, competencies and abilities, as well as a clear indication of potential development.

Figure 1.1 illustrates the types of material from which a personal portfolio collection might be constructed.

Types of personal portfolio material

Each one of our lives is unique and our individual personal portfolios should reflect this uniqueness.

For example, I have a friend who left school at sixteen with two 'O' levels. She then did a variety of jobs, including shop assistant, garage forecourt attendant, domestic help and package-tour courier, before embarking upon a nursing career. After a career break to raise a family, she returned to nursing as a part-timer and then qualified as a tutor. She went on to do research and gained a PhD. Currently, she occupies her time and earns her keep by writing novels. Every aspect of her life has shaped her identity and her work. Table 1.1 contains a

Figure 1.1 Types of Personal Portfolio Material

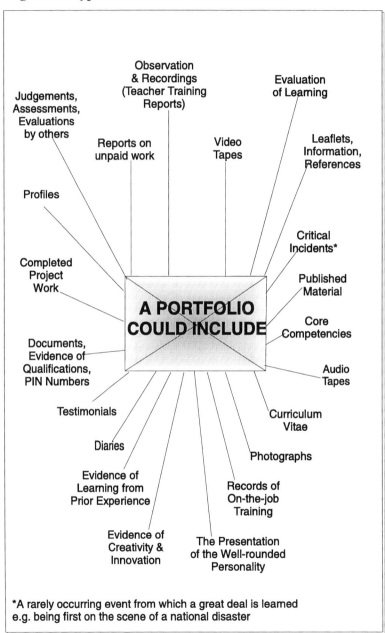

list of suggested sources from which your personal portfolio might be constructed.

Table 1.1: Origins of personal portfolio evidence

1. Professional preparation and development
   a) Statutory qualifications
   b) Recordable qualifications
   c) Short courses and study days
   d) In service training days

2. Education
   a) School leaving qualifications
   b) Higher education
      i) Certificate level
      ii) Diploma level
      iii) Degree level
      iv) Post-graduate level
   c) Other

3. Paid employment
   a) Professional work
   b) Consultancy
   c) Publications, conferences
   d) Projects

4. Voluntary Work
   a) Public services
   b) Charities
   c) Fund raising

5. Leisure activities
   a) Sport
   b) Hobbies and craftwork

c)   Learning new skills

d)   Outside interests

6.   Family and domestic life

a)   Child rearing

b)   Household management

c)   Catering

7.   You as a person

a)   How you present yourself both on paper and personally

b)   How you relate to others

The comprehensiveness of your personal portfolio means that it is essentially a personal and, therefore, private collection of your biographical data, which should be controlled by you and remain your property. No other person has right of access to the information contained in your personal portfolio. How it is organised and structured is a matter for your personal preference. The guiding principle should be that it is easy for you to use.

Having firmly established that the personal portfolio is the private property of the author, we need now to consider how selected elements of this material become public in the form of a profile.

Personal profiles

For the purposes of this book, a profile is defined in the following way:

> *'A collection of evidence which is selected from the personal portfolio for a particular purpose and for the attention of a particular audience.'*

At this point, the elements of the personal portfolio selected to construct the profile cease to be private because they are being specifically prepared for public release to a particular audience. Therefore, you, as the author of the profile, cease to be the exclusive owner of the information. What was once a private collection now becomes a public display! At the same time, certain ethical issues become important in relation to the rights and obligations of you, the owner of the information, and to those of the audience with whom you have shared it. The issue of confidentiality influences the kind of information which is disclosed, and how appropriate the disclosure is in relation to the reasons for its release.

Example:

If you are applying for the post of an equal opportunities officer, you may decide to select critical incidents from your own life to illustrate your knowledge of the inequality experienced by others. By drawing on personal experience, you could illustrate how you identified the inequality, your analysis of its underlying causes and how these were handled. This kind of evidence might be said to be inappropriately disclosed if you are applying for a post with a different focus.

Table 1.2: Advantages of personal portfolio/profile development to the nurse

Professional/education development

- ⌘ Facilitates periodic registration and update (UKCC)
- ⌘ Enables the effectiveness of Post Registration Education and Practice (PREP)
- ⌘ Offers progression as a Professional, Specialist and Advanced Practitioner
- ⌘ Conforms to the Framework for Continuing Professional Education (ENB)
- ⌘ Offers the opportunity for indexing for the Higher Award (ENB)
- ⌘ Facilitates the operation of the Credit Accumulation and Transfer System (CATS)
- ⌘ Facilitates credit exemption which is cost effective and reduces the duplication of learning
- ⌘ May facilitate access to courses of study with advanced standing

⌘ Promotes your contribution towards quality assurance

⌘ Enhances your professional performance for the benefit of clients

Career development

⌘ Can facilitate the identification of your training needs and goals

⌘ Gives opportunities for self-evaluation and reflection

⌘ Gives a systematic review of your past and current achievements, learning and contributions to quality care

⌘ Contributes towards your staff appraisal or individual performance review

⌘ Demonstrates the appropriateness of your individual characteristics in relation to a particular job specification

⌘ Can be used to construct a *curriculum vitae* (CV) or complete an application form

⌘ Can be used as evidence at job interviews or to develop a presentation to a panel

⌘ Facilitates a return to professional practice after a career break

Personal development

⌘ Can facilitate a change of direction in your career

⌘ Encourages you to acknowledge and apply your life skills to your work and vice versa

⌘ Encourages your self-assessment and insight

⌘ Builds your self-confidence and enhances motivation

⌘ Maximises your potential

⌘ Facilitates your return to paid employment after a career break

Table 1.2 gives some examples of the advantages and purposes for which personal portfolios, and the subsequent profiles which are developed from them, can be used. These advantages may be extended to other agencies with whom you have contact, such as employing authorities (see Table 1.3) and the training agencies they use. The advantages to employing authorities are significant in economic terms. Used effectively, portfolios can make important contributions to staff development and training, because they can help nurse educators to develop courses which are specifically tailored to meet staff and client needs.

Table 1.3: Advantages of personal portfolio/profile development to other agencies

To Employers:

⌘ A means of ensuring that there is a match between the job and person specification match

⌘ Promotes effective recruitment procedures

⌘ Facilitates a mutually beneficial Individual Performance Review procedure

⌘ Enhances staff confidence and progression

⌘ Promotes analysis of job satisfaction and can reduce staff wastage

⌘ Reduces duplication of training/education programmes

⌘ Facilitates identification of training needs

⌘ Contributes towards the maintenance of quality assurance

To Education/Training Organisations

⌘ A means of increasing the appropriateness of education/training provision to students' needs

⌘ Ensures that the educational/training provision has the capacity to maintain and improve standards of care to the public

⌘ Facilitates the operation of CATS and APEL

⌘ Promotes the quality of provision using flexible modes of delivery

⌘ Facilitates the identification of new student groups

A personal portfolio needs to have the following qualities (see Table 1.4)

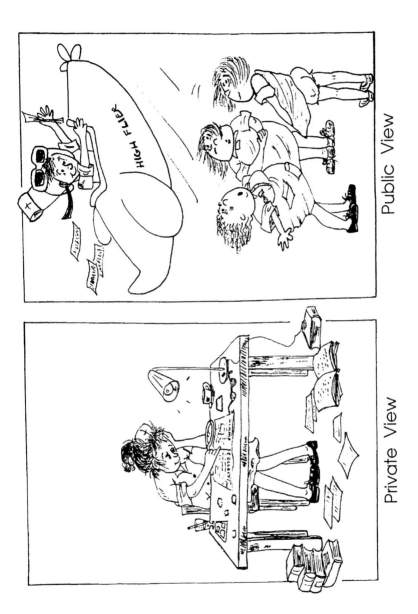

Public View

Private View

Table 1.4: Qualities of a personal portfolio

Flexible	Accessible
Comprehensive	Well-presented
Well-organised	Up-to-date
Versatile	Accurate
Concise	Lucid
Manageable	Relevant

If your personal portfolio has these qualities, it is more likely that the profiles, which you construct from it, will do the job they are supposed to do.

The storage and organisation of material

Where you keep your material and how you organise it is important; it must be both accessible to you and organised in such a way that is useful to you. Your organisation of it must be one that you understand and will enjoy using.

For example, leaving your personal portfolio collection at your mother's home in the Isle of Man is not a good idea unless you work there. If you keep your portfolio in the attic, the chances are that you will not go to the trouble of keeping it up-to-date.

If you are not comfortable with computers, it would be unwise to transfer the collection on to a disk. However, you might like to consider the acquisition of word-processing skills as part of your future development!

Your portfolio is unlikely to be confined to written records. You may need to organise collections of photographic or video materials. Figure 1.1 illustrates the diversity of sources for personal portfolio material. An A4 ring binder with clearly titled sections might be a useful starting point. Additional material could be kept in well-organised box files or in a small filing cabinet.

Several packages are now available which provide helpful models on how to organise your material. You can modify them to suit your own individual needs. These include the Welsh National Board Professional Profile (similar to a personal organiser), the profile pack

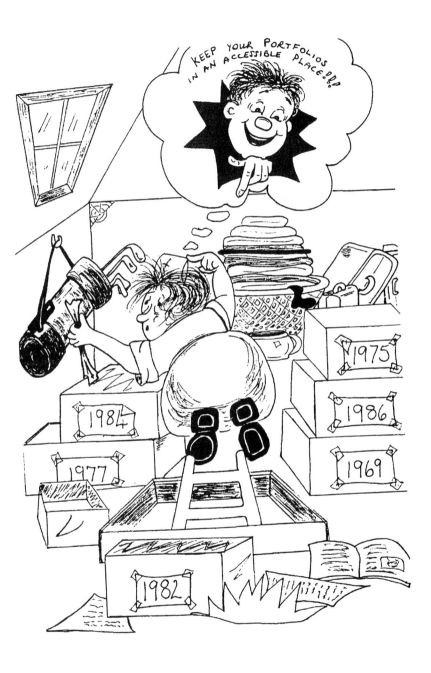

published by Macmillan for the Nursing Times (1993), and the Professional Portfolio published by the English National Board (1991) (note the different titles used for similar publications). A detailed evaluation of some commonly available packages is contained in Chapter 7.

You may *have* to use one of these packages. For example, should you wish to become indexed with the English National Board for the Higher Award, you will be required to purchase and use the ENB Professional Portfolio for documenting your professional development. This publication can provide a valuable recording device for your collection but you may need to supplement it with additional material. For example, the section on assessment for specific credits for **prior learning** (APL) requires the signature of your assessor to confirm how many credits you have achieved and how you have achieved them. Your assessor will require evidence that you have achieved the learning outcomes, which could include project work, supervised practice, or evidence of innovation.

In the following chapters, there will be an outline of the initial creation of a **personal portfolio**, and then an examination of the construction of specific **profiles** for particular tasks. These will include periodic registration, indexing for the ENB Higher Award, registration as a Specialist Practitioner and application for courses in higher education.

I hope this introductory chapter has been helpful in making the important distinction between **personal portfolios** and **profiles**, despite the confusion which may continue to arise in relation to the various terms used by different authorities. You may still be asked by an educational establishment to provide a portfolio assisting in, for example, a **credit rating** exercise, in order for you to embark upon an academic course of study. Select the appropriate material from your **personal portfolio** to enable the completion of this task. It should not be necessary, and may indeed be unethical, for you to be required to send the whole contents. Most institutions provide helpful guidelines regarding their requirements. This will be discussed in more detail in Chapter 6.

Chapter 2

Creating your personal portfolio from your *Curriculum Vitae*

In the previous chapter, there was a definition of the terms and an outline of the advantages aimed at nurses and other agencies of the personal portfolio and profiles. The storage, management and maintenance of the portfolio have also been addressed.

In this chapter, how to begin the process of creating your own personal portfolio will be considered.

The extended *curriculum vitae*

A useful starting point for this is to write out a detailed, extended *curriculum vitae* (CV). Rebecca Corfield (1990) defines a CV as '.. *an outline of a person's educational and professional history.'*

How you organise your extended *curriculum vitae* depends on your own personal preference and the format that you find most useful. You may find the headings used in Figure 2.1 (overleaf) helpful to begin with. The core headings are generally applicable to most people. The optional headings can be used if they are appropriate for you personally or, alternatively, you can create some different headings.

Additionally, you should include some personal details at the beginning of the CV, if only to identify it as yours. This includes most of the information required on the front page of the majority of application forms (see Table 2.1).

Figure 2.1: *Curriculum Vitae* Core Headings and Options

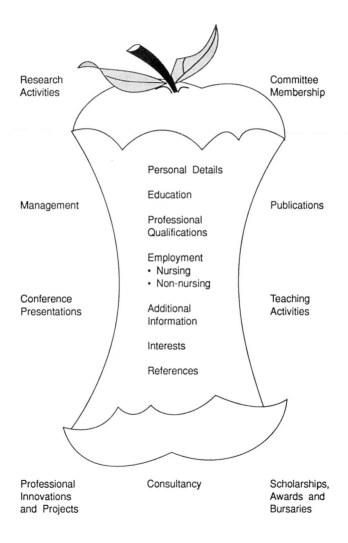

Research
Activities

Committee
Membership

Management

Publications

Personal Details

Education

Professional
Qualifications

Employment
• Nursing
• Non-nursing

Conference
Presentations

Teaching
Activities

Additional
Information

Interests

References

Professional
Innovations
and Projects

Consultancy

Scholarships,
Awards and
Bursaries

Table 2.1: Personal information

Surname	Forename(s)	Age
Title	Address (home)	Date of birth
Work telephone no.		Marital status*
Home telephone no.		Present post
PIN number		Present employer
Number and ages* of dependants		Current salary/scale
Ethnic group*		Current driving licence
*see p12, 13		

It is worth reminding ourselves at this point that the CV will form the core of a portfolio which is personal and private to you in the first instance. You may not always wish to use some of the information contained in this in relation to particular functions or activities. For example, if an employer has an equal opportunities policy, information regarding number of dependants, marital status and ethnicity may not be required. However, an organisation may have a system of monitoring its equal opportunities policy by the collection of such information. If so, this can be collected separately by the Personnel Department, if you agree to provide it.

The personal details which you include in your personal portfolio should serve only as an *aide memoire*. The appropriate selection of what to include, or otherwise, when you extract your data for a particular purpose, is your decision.

A typical extended CV may contain headings as indicated in the left-hand column in Table 2.2. You may compare this with the headings that I use in my CV developed specifically for my work in higher education (see right hand column). This example also illustrates that different headings may be more suitable according to the type of career that you have led. For instance, a specialist nurse with a high level of expertise in a particular clinical area may need to include a section on 'Innovations in Practice' or 'Research Activities'.

Table 2.2: *curriculum vitae* **contents**

Standard	Specific
Personal information	Personal details
General education (Secondary/Further/Higher)	Academic/professional qualifications
Professional recordable qualifications*	Present post
Professional non-recordable qualifications (courses, study days, etc.)*	Previous posts
Current post	Research interests/course planning activities
Previous nursing employment (starting with the most recent)	Academic activities
Previous non-nursing employment	Professional activities
Unpaid work experience	Published work
Interests (hobbies, leisure activities)	Consultancy
Additional information	Conference papers presented
References	Other activities
*see Glossary, p94	

It is often useful to include in your extended CV a section which is headed 'Other Information and Activities'. This can sometimes lead to you making a new heading which is quite specific. Some of these activities may have quite a few areas in common (a fact which you may not appreciate until you list them). For example, you may feel that you have not published a great deal until you include this activity under the 'Other Information' heading. You may then discover that you have had published several items which are worthy of putting in their own individual category headed 'Publications'.

You might like to include at the end of your CV the names, titles, addresses and telephone numbers of people who would be suitable and willing current referees for you. These could relate to different areas of your life. For example, I include individuals who have knowledge of my performance in terms of my:

⌘ academic life   ⌘ work in the NHS

⌘ research activities   ⌘ charitable work

These, along with the other information in your CV, will need periodic updating. Figure 2.1 illustrates the core headings that most CVs will generate, along with some optional themes that may arise from individual careers. Try to put as much information as you can in your extended CV at this point.

When compiling your extended CV it is well worth the effort of considering carefully the layout, organisation and consistency of your presentation. For instance, it is useful to keep to capital letters for major headings; to record events in date order with the most recent first, if appropriate; to use an acknowledged reference system (e.g. Harvard, British Standard BS 5605:1990) when recording publications. See example below:

PUBLICATIONS

BROWN, R A (1989). *Individualised Care: The Role of the Ward Sister.* Scutari Publications, Harrow.

BROWN, R A (1995). Education for specialist and advanced practice. *Br J Nurs*, **4**:5.

It is likely that your extended CV will run into several pages. If this is so, you may like to consider using different coloured paper for major sections (blue pages for post-registration professional development, for example). If you do this, don't forget to construct a contents list and a code at the beginning. The development of your extended CV is a task that you can begin immediately. It is then ready to use when you decide on the particular route that your career is to take. For example, if you decide to index for the ENB Higher Award you will be able to use the information that you have collected so far to begin the process of compiling the ENB Professional Portfolio.

An abridged *curriculum vitae*

The completion of your extended CV is a major step in the development of your portfolio. Once you have completed this task, you may like to consider using selected information to create an abridged version of your CV to include in support of job applications, etc. It should not be longer than two A4 pages and be appropriate for public disclosure of your details. Corfield (1990) provides some useful examples of alternative approaches to completing this task and also highlights some of the advantages of having an abridged version of your CV available at all times.

Appendix 1 contains a fictional abridged CV of a nurse who qualified in 1988. She has recently started work as a junior sister.

Chapter 3

Enhancing the headings: From CV to Portfolio

Once you have taken the first step of creating your curriculum vitae, it is useful to go through it and flesh out this outline of your life to date. You can use the existing documentary evidence that you already have. This evidence should confirm what you have done, and also provide documentation about what you have learned from what you did. You should also be able to say how this contributed towards your personal and professional development. Most important of all, you should be able to say how the learning experience enabled you to contribute to both maintaining and improving the quality of client care.

Personal details

Look first at your personal details; this will lead you to gather together a collection of valuable personal documents which confirm your personal identity. Examples of these are included in Table 3.1. As these documents are so valuable in their original form, it is worth considering keeping two copies of each in your personal portfolio (one as a master copy—the other to use when required as supporting documentation). Do not be tempted to release original documents unless specifically requested. Should an agency require sight of an original document, either deal with it in person and stay with the documents, or ensure that a named person in the receiving organisation accepts responsibility for the safe keeping of your document. In this case, always use recorded postal delivery to a designated person.

Table 3.1: Personal identity documentation

Birth certificate	Work permit
Marriage certificate	Deed poll (name changes)
Certification of disability	Driving licence
UKCC PIN No & card	NHS card
Trade Union membership card	

It is also worth considering keeping a set of up-to-date passport photographs of yourself in this section of your database. These are sometimes requested in relation to different profiles which could be required of you. Similarly, you will also have available evidence of your Professional Identification Number (PIN) from the UKCC. This will be supplied to you at initial and subsequent periodic registration in the form of a plastic card similar to a credit card. I have found it useful to file this evidence in the following way:

- ⌘ The signed plastic receipt card is stored with my credit cards so that it is kept safely and is readily available

- ⌘ The PIN number is recorded in the personal details section on my extended CV and in the data section of my personal organiser/diary

- ⌘ The backing sheet which accompanied the card is retained and I write the expiry date of the card on this and store with the other documents in my portfolio

The backing sheet which comes with your card is a useful reminder about the management of your PIN card and the address of the UKCC (see Appendix 2).

You might also like to include in this section your first salary slip for each new incremental year that you enter. This will not only help you to keep track of your salary progression, but can also be used to provide potential new employers with information about your current salary level.

General education

Documentary evidence in this section can be organised in a variety of ways. You might like to think about those categories depicted in Table 3.2. The organisation of this area of your portfolio needs careful thinking through. You may need to cross-reference between the higher and professional education sections as there could be considerable overlap between these two.

Table 3.2: Organisation of formal educational evidence

GENERAL	
Primary	School reports
Secondary	School reports, copies of certificates
Higher	Projects, reports, certificates, diplomas, degrees
Post-graduate	Dissertations, higher degrees, projects
PROFESSIONAL	
Pre-registration	RGN. RMN. RNMH. RM. RN (Adult) BSc (Hons) Nursing, RGN/RMN
Post-registration	Certificate in Education Diploma in Community Nursing DPSN/BSc (Hons) Nursing Studies English National Board validated courses Statutory updating

Beginning with the primary education experience, it may only be necessary to identify where and when you attended school, between the ages of five and eleven, in both your extended and abridged CV. However, you may feel that there was something exceptional about your primary school experience. This might be in relation to its location or its approach to the curriculum, (it took place in the Solomon Islands or it used a Montessori approach in terms of free expression). You might, then, like to write a short account of how this important early experience influenced your later development, philosophy and practice. You may not have given yourself the opportunity to do this in the past and it may help your development as a reflective individual.

Supporting documentary evidence in relation to your secondary school experience may take the form of copies of certificates gained (e.g. GCSE, 'A' level) and school reports. A short account of significant events could be included at this point. You may have been a prefect or captain of the hockey team. Extra curricular activities are also worth remembering, such as obtaining sponsorship to attend an Outward Bound course or undertaking a European tour with the County Youth Orchestra. If your school days are further back than you care to remember, a record in your CV of dates, place of education and qualifications gained will be sufficient. Other, later experiences will take greater prominence and your most recent memories are more likely to allow you to develop your portfolio information base.

Higher and professional education

For this section, you will need to consider how you organise your evidence in relation to your higher and professional education, as there is considerable blurring between the two areas. This is particularly so in relation to the development of Project 2000 and the conjoint validation of both pre- and post-registration courses.

My own rule of thumb for such dilemmas is that any documentary evidence for qualifications which relate to my work as a nurse, whether statutory or otherwise (e.g. RGN, Diploma in Nursing, DPSN), would be filed firstly in the Professional Education category. However, I would make a secondary reference to such things as the Diploma in Nursing in the Higher Education (HE) section, as well as inserting duplicate copies of documents, if this were not too expensive. My reasoning for doing this would be the recognition/validation of the qualification by an academic institution rather than by a statutory body (ENB).

If the qualification has been jointly validated by a National Board and a higher education institution, such as a university/college of HE (as is the case with most Project 2000 courses which also offer a Diploma), the same principle could apply (see Appendix 1).

An Open University degree in the social sciences and a pre-Project 2000 RNMH pose no problems using this system. The documentation for the degree is entered in the higher education file, and the RNMH information in the Professional Education section.

The evidence for both higher and professional education is likely to be very similar and takes the form of copies of certificates, diplomas, degrees and registration documents. Careful documentation of other registration numbers, besides those pertaining to the UKCC, should be made. For example, most nurse tutors who have a Certificate of Education are registered as teachers with the Department of Education and Science, as well as with the UKCC as Registered Nurse Tutors.

Copies of major projects of a good standard can also be included, as can records of course work reports, examination marks, and any credits and distinctions gained. Copies of assessed work on a course that you are currently undertaking can be invaluable. I recently interviewed a student who was undertaking a Diploma course in another part of the country and who wished to transfer, in the middle of the academic year, to the university where I work. It would have been very difficult to arrive at a fair and just decision had she not been able to provide me with information about her course. This included copies of the course work that she had completed to date, a syllabus of the course she was currently undertaking, and a report of her progress from her course tutor. (Further discussion of this kind of issue will be undertaken in the chapter on Credit Accumulation and Transfer, as will verification by self and others). It is vital that the following dimensions are clear from this information:

1. That learning took place as a consequence of these studies;

2. That this learning enabled you to both maintain and develop your contribution to high quality client care.

Although it is tempting to squirrel away everything but the kitchen sink, it is worth putting a time limit on how long you store materials such as course work. It should certainly be kept for the duration of the course itself and perhaps for 2–5 years following completion, depending on your storage circumstances. Most pieces of work carry a critique and grade from the marker. This could be retained when the work is finally discarded. Failing this, you could complete a short synopsis of the work that you did and the standard achieved, for future reference.

Some evidence of course content should be noted. Course information leaflets can usually be relied upon to provide a brief résumé of the course outline, length, mode of attendance and assessment. Student handbooks usually provide a more detailed account of course content.

Additional educational experience

Additional educational experience may include any other educational activities, which do not fit neatly under the major headings already discussed and summarised in Table 3.2. Again, it may be helpful to set up further categories, according to the different activities that you have engaged in to date. Initially, you might like to sit and write a list covering everything from in-service study days to Local Authority Evening Classes. These could then be put in some kind of order, before you decide about the kind of supporting documentation which you either already have available or can obtain from other sources. Table 3.3 illustrates some of the options which you might like to consider when organising sections in your portfolio for your additional informal educational experience.

Table 3.3: Organisation of informal educational evidence

	Activities undertaken	Supporting evidence
Professional	In-service study In-service courses Conferences attended	Evidence of attendance Programmes Summarise what you have learned and whether this influences your professional performance, e.g. a list of competencies
Voluntary work training	Samaritans Rape Crisis or Relate counsellor Justice of the Peace etc.	As above. Document how this enhances your professional performance. Testimonials

	Activities undertaken	**Supporting evidence**
Supplementary	Courses on word processing, public speaking	The presentation of your CV and your verbal performance at an interview are opportunities to provide evidence
Non-vocational	Interest and skill-based adult education classes, such as upholstery, local history	Evidence of manual dexterity—items you have made, photographs etc.
Leisure activities	Bell ringing, bird watching, fell walking. May include independent, self-directed study	Write about your own development in relation to teamwork, observation skills and stamina

The overviews of both formal and informal educational experiences contained in Tables 3.2 and 3.3 clearly indicate that the evidence for each of them comes from two different sources. The first is primary evidence, which is either produced by you in the form of essays, articles, course work, projects, etc., and the other is secondary evidence, which comes from other people. This evidence is usually in the form of official acknowledgement of your successful completion of some form of study or activity e.g. academic awards, prizes and testimonials. Table 3.4 summarises the categories of evidence in relation to where they come from.

Table 3.4: Categories of evidence

Primary (produced by the individual)	**Secondary** (produced by others)	
	Collective (on behalf of an institution)	**Individual** (usually the view of one person)
Projects, Published Works, Artefacts, Photographs, Video/Audio Recordings, Essays	Prizes, Bursaries, Scholarships, Academic Awards	Reports, Testimonials, Reviews

When collecting together your supporting evidence for activities which you have undertaken, ask yourself:

> *"How can I best convey to others what I have learned from this activity?"*

> *"Is this sufficient proof to support the learning that I have achieved and the quality of care that I give?"*

> *"How can I show the effect of this learning on the quality of care that I give?"*

Do not be overcome by modesty—what you have learned is invaluable. In the first instance, it has to be valued by you, in order for it to be valued by others. You must use every opportunity offered to you to demonstrate its value.

Current post

It should not be too difficult to provide evidence for your portfolio relating to your present job. A useful starting point, which you could include, is your current job description. This should illustrate the skills which you needed to bring to this job and which you clearly had or you would not have been appointed. Following that, you need to show how you have developed both the job and yourself. This could include documentation of innovations which you have introduced and evaluated in your area of work. If you have failed to document them, perhaps you would like to pause for a moment and reflect on why you did not do this. Perhaps this task could become one of your goals for the future. The innovations in which you may have been involved could include one or some of the following:

- ⌘ the introduction and monitoring of primary nursing
- ⌘ the organisation of a journal club
- ⌘ the preparation and management of a mentorship system for learners
- ⌘ the development of a support network for a particular client group

Additionally, you may have become an expert in a particular area of client care, such as tissue viability, diabetes, terminal illness... —the list is endless (most qualified nurses are experts in some specific area or other— if you're not, maybe you could reflect also on why this is!) You may have shared your experience by writing articles, preparing patient guidelines, developing philosophies of care or speaking at conferences, study days or seminars. Where documentary evidence is non-existent, try to obtain some evaluation of what you did from one of your secondary sources (see Table 3.4). For example, if you have presented a seminar paper, you could ask for some evaluation from the organiser and/or the audience. Conference papers are sometimes published and there may be reports of conference proceedings in periodicals etc. It is unlikely that you will need the services of a press cuttings agency at this point, but you never know!

Finally, if you don't find reflection on your everyday work life easy, you might like to consider keeping a diary record of your job for one week. You can then use this to analyse your professional activities, particularly in terms of what you have learned and how you have used your new knowledge.

Previous nursing employment

The work that you did in previous appointments needs to be summarised. The job description, if you still have it, can be used as the core material, with supporting evidence in précis form. This should illustrate how you were able to develop the role and what you learned from the experience. In a nutshell, this means what you did for the job and what the job did for you. Additionally, you might like to include testimonials from your senior managers—if this is possible—along with other material which is suggested in the section relating to your current job.

Non-nursing employment (paid and unpaid)

It is important to document any other work that you have done. Again, how you categorise this depends on your own personal preference and circumstances. One suggestion is to use a heading '**Non-nursing Work**' and subdivide it into **paid** and **unpaid employment**. You could include voluntary and domestic work in the latter if you wish. The same principles used to document your previous nursing experience could apply in this section, i.e. record where, when and what you did. Supplement this with evidence that both you and others have generated, to indicate what you were able to do and what you learned. Highlight the enhancement of existing competencies and the development of new ones. Try not to undervalue unpaid work. Caring for elderly relatives, managing the domestic life of a family or organising a mail order club require skills of a high order. What you need is the evidence to substantiate that you have done them and learned from your experience. Younger colleagues will need to emphasise part-time work done, perhaps during the last years at school. Being able to carry out a paper round requires a degree of dependability, stamina, tenacity, a muscular left shoulder and a well-organised approach. This last Christmas was my son's first time carrying out such an activity. The number of Christmas 'tips' that he received gave me some indication of how effective he was at this job. People would not have responded in this way if he tended to be late, absent, delivering to the wrong address, etc.. However, I must advise against you recording in your portfolio your annual receipt of chocolates, sherry, silk stockings, theatre tickets, etc.. from grateful clients, but there is a moral (or two) there somewhere! There is also a subtle difference between measuring people's appreciation of what you do and the skills that you learn from doing it. That is not to say that the clients' view of what you do is unimportant. Perhaps this is an opportune moment to reflect on what constitutes good practice and who defines it!

Voluntary work

This area of your life may embrace more formal types of voluntary work, such as being a Justice of the Peace, which should pose no problems in terms of documentation. Less formal types of voluntary work are also valid to record in relation to developing competencies.

This may include youth club work, fund raising for charity, etc.. Some time ago I organised a flower festival at a local church. I have kept records such as the accounts, the programme of events, press cuttings and photographs. I also took the unprecedented step of asking for a budget of six hundred pounds. This was a high-risk request for all sorts of reasons (not least because, in normal circumstances, the cash flow is in the opposite direction). The good news is that there was a 100% return on the outlay. Even better news (with an eye to the outcomes), was the fact that many people gained a great deal of pleasure from this event. It also provided the fulcrum for releasing talents and strengthening interpersonal relationships and, thus, the enhancement of team building.

Leisure activities

What we do with our spare time gives valuable insights to others about the kind of people we are, in terms of what motivates and enthuses us. It can also highlight those areas of our professional lives which we would like to develop more.

In my own life, I have enjoyed being with others and sharing experiences and ideas with them. Initially, I had to make a conscious effort to overcome a basic shyness. Joining several evening classes in pottery helped me to forget my self-consciousness as I pursued learning a new skill. Eventually, I became more confident in groups. Those early experiences helped me, at work, to relate to strangers, whether new colleagues or clients, and undoubtedly contributed to my ability to work as a teacher later on.

Additional information

Your portfolio may contain any items and supporting documentation which do not naturally fit into those areas already discussed. The content may well change over time, as your career develops. It is possible that, early on, you may not have engaged in a consultancy role. At some point this may be worthy of a brief mention and later become more significant as this role develops, so as to require a section dedicated to this area of your work.

You should now have available to you a significant database on which you can draw to produce profiles for a variety of purposes. In the next chapters, there will be an examination of specific issues in relation to profiling for the National Boards and the UKCC. Additionally, the use of the profile for accessing Higher Education courses using CATS (Credit Accumulation and Transfer System) and APL (Assessment of Prior Learning) will be considered.

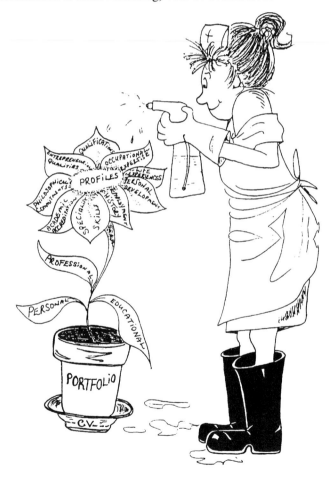

Big profiles out of little CVs grow

Chapter 4

Goal setting and profiles for periodic registration

The previous chapters concentrated on the construction of your CV (abridged and extended), which was then developed, by the addition of supporting documentation, into a personal portfolio. This demonstrated what you had gained from the experiences you described and indicated how you used your learning to improve your professional performance as a nurse. The work done so far will have given you a clear overview of your achievements to date and enabled you to identify and reflect on areas of your life, both professional and personal, that you would like to develop.

Personal and professional goals

The next important phase of your personal portfolio development is the creation of a section which looks to the future and enables you to set personal and professional goals. You may not have consciously done this in the past. However, if you are to undertake your professional development effectively, this activity will be most important. The type of goals that you set will probably fall into two categories:

1.   Those that you set for yourself
2.   Those that are negotiated with, or imposed by, other individuals or organisations

Figure 4.1 (overleaf) illustrates examples of some of the goals you or others might identify. They will differ according to the kind of work you do, the nature of the career you wish to pursue and the kind of life you live.

Obviously, some goals will take longer than others to achieve. Some will need to be addressed immediately, e.g. those relating to punctuality, arranging a meeting with your boss for your appraisal interview and chairing a meeting the following day. Table 4.1 illustrates goal categories in relation to time spans.

Figure 4.1: Goal setting

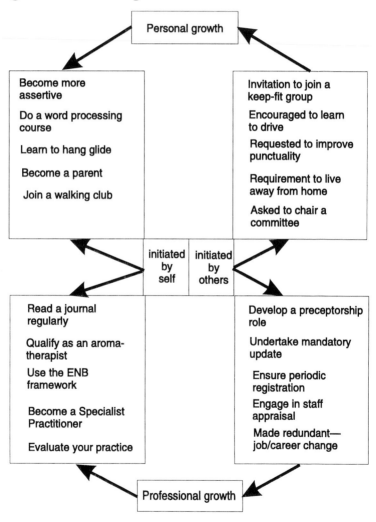

Table 4.1: Goal categories in terms of time span

Immediate	Improve punctuality Read a journal regularly Write an extended CV
Short-term (achievable in six months)	Attend a conference on the ENB framework Undertake a course in study skills Learn to drive and buy a car
Medium-term (achievable in one year)	Become more assertive Complete ENB 870 course (or equivalent module at level 2) Write an article on individualised care
Long-term (achievable in longer than one year)	Become a specialist practitioner Do a post-registration degree Fulfil periodic registration requirements

It is useful to note in your portfolio, not only your goals, but also how you are going to achieve them and how you will judge your success. It is important to estimate how long it will take to achieve your goals. A good habit would be to review your goal section annually—a creative New Year's resolution perhaps! Then you could check off the things you have achieved and insert them in the appropriate section of your portfolio. You could also review the progress of your long-term goals and make changes if necessary. To complete your review, you will need to identify new goals, and document the things you did that were unplanned (and, therefore, an unexpected bonus). If you discover that you have amassed more than several such windfalls, while at the same time not achieving many of the goals you originally set for yourself, I suggest you have cause to reflect:

⌘ Are you sufficiently focused in your efforts?

⌘ Are you avoiding the achievement of your objectives and, if so, why?

⌘ What external influences are preventing you from achieving your goals?

⌘ Are you able to take action about these?

If your achievements pertain predominantly to either your professional or your private life, I would also encourage you to reflect on the fact that in order to become consistently productive and happy, well-rounded personalities, we need to attend to both work and leisure interests.

Verification

Our discussions so far have implied that there should be some sort of formal **verification** or **confirmation** that we have learned what we say we have learned. This proof can come from a variety of sources from either yourself or others, as shown by the evidence discussed in Chapter 3, which included suggestions for the documentation of your previous experience (e.g. diplomas, testimonials).The ENB Professional Portfolio contains a section for other experiences which can be used to obtain accreditation under an assessment of prior learning (APL) system. The format the ENB have developed indicates that you should supply proof of prior learning which must also be assessed or verified by an assessor.

UKCC requirements

The UKCC (1994) on the other hand, is mainly concerned with the maintenance of an effective registration by the fulfilment of four statutory requirements. These include the completion of a profile and they are as follows:

⌘ completion of five study days every three years

⌘ completion of a Notification of Practice form every three years

⌘ completion of a Return to Practice programme if you have had a break in practice of five years or more

⌘ maintenance of details of professional development in a personal professional profile

Five day of study

The requirement for a minimum of five days of study means just that. Many nurses are worried about what this will actually entail in terms of study leave (paid or unpaid), extra travel to study centres and expensive fees. What the UKCC really require is that practitioners engage in a variety of learning activities throughout their professional lives. The Council have identified five areas of study which offer a number of possibilities. These five areas are listed below with some examples of the kind of learning activity that would be appropriate:

⌘ **Patient, client & colleague support**
Counselling, leadership, networking, mentorship skills

e.g. plan and develop a satellite ant natal clinic for Asian women with colleagues

⌘ **Care enhancement**
New approaches to care
Quality assurance
Health promotion/education

e.g. review the literature in relation to men's health and set up a well man's clinic

⌘ **Practice development**
Evaluate service provision
Personal research in your area of practice

e.g. organise some teaching sessions from the clinical nurse specialist for you and your team

⌘ **Reducing risk**
Identify health problems
Evaluate your health education/promotion role

e.g. complete a study module on teaching and learning skills

⌘ **Education development**
Exchange visits with centres of excellence
Attend a conference/seminar/workshop
Join a journal club

e.g. earmark some of your budget for 1–2 journal subscriptions for your area and begin a monthly journal club

These learning activities must be relevant to your current area of work and you need to plan and document your study activity carefully. A good example of this is to keep a record of the reading that you do and how you critique and use this knowledge in practice. Your professional profile is ideal for doing this, so that you can extract the relevant information when you come to re-register. The Council will require you to keep these records for a minimum of six years, as well as self-verifying what you have learned and how. You will need to do this from 1 April 1998 when you apply to renew your registration. This will take the form of a formal declaration from you that you have fulfilled your statutory obligations in relation to the minimum requirement of five study days or their equivalent every three years. This is to ensure that you have maintained your professional development and that you have the appropriate level of competence for the area in which you work. The UKCC (1995) are quite clear that:

> '...*you, the individual practitioner, are ultimately responsible for ensuring you fulfil your professional obligations and renew your registration.*' *Fact Sheet 5*

The UKCC intend to set up an audit system to monitor and evaluate how this operates. This will officially begin after the 31 March 2001. In the meantime, the Council will carry out pilot studies in order to arrive at the final format for this procedure.

Notification of Practice

From 1 April 1995, you will need to complete a Notification of Practice form in the following circumstances:

⌘ every three years when you apply to renew your registration

⌘ if you change your area of practice to one in which you need to use a different registrable qualification

⌘ if you return to practice after a break of five years or more.

This form, which the UKCC will send to you, will require information about your practice, such as:

⌘ whether you are full- or part-time

⌘ the location of your practice, e.g. theatres, community or intensive care

⌘ who your employers are, e.g. general practitioner fund holders, residential home or hospital trust

⌘ the qualification that you are currently using for your practice.

This information will provide a valuable data base about the number of nurses working in a variety of specialisms and for a variety of employers. It will also provide the first ever comprehensive profile of the qualified nursing labour force in the UK since registration began in 1919. Used judiciously, it could become a powerful tool in the formulation of arguments about skill mix, education/training provision and the redeployment of staff in response to epidemiological trends.

Your Notification of Practice is a legal requirement. This means that if you do not complete the Notification of Practice form, your registration will not be renewed and you will be unable to engage in professional practice.

Return to professional practice

There are additional statutory requirements in relation to your return to professional practice following a career break or a change in area of practice of five years or more. The Council are quite specific about what a break in service means in terms of the minimum amount spent in practice. If you have worked for less than 100 days (a day can be interpreted as one regular session) or 750 hours during the previous five years, this constitutes a break in practice. You will, therefore, need to undertake a 'return to practice' programme and successfully complete an assessment of your competence, which must be recorded and verified in your profile. You could, at the same time, complete the section on your short-, medium- and long-term professional goals. Additionally, you should keep a careful record of the time that you spend in practice and the work that you do. You can use your profile to store this information.

The Personal Professional Profile

The Personal Professional Profile that the UKCC will require you to keep is a record of your career progress and your professional development. Fact sheet 4 in the UKCC's information pack (1995) states that your profile has two important functions:

⌘ it will contribute to your professional development by helping you to recognise, understand and value your abilities, strengths, achievements and experience

⌘ it provides a source of information upon which you can draw at any time and if required to do so by the UKCC for the purpose of compiling information about standards of education following registration

This could be the first, most important, profile you extract from your personal portfolio. It will demonstrate whether you are a fit and proper person to continue your working life as a professional nurse. This is really the first time since the Nurses Act of 1919, that you have been made personally responsible and accountable in terms of your rights to remain a practitioner. In the past, once you had become registered, you were able to practise for life (unless you were reported for misconduct to the statutory body and subsequently struck off). This will no longer be the case. The buck will stop with your personal profile, so it is crucial that you get it right. You will probably need guidance and support to do this. If you are a newly qualified practitioner, you should be able to obtain this from your allocated **preceptor**. However, because it is the first time that this kind of support has been formally included in policy, you may have to give these developments a little time to be implemented.

The provision of support

The Council's commitment to the role of preceptor is encapsulated in the following statement:

> `The Council considers that, as good practice, all newly registered nurses, midwives and health visitors should be provided with a period of support, where possible under the guidance of a preceptor, for approximately the first four months of registered practice.'
>
> UKCC (1995) Registrar's Letter, 3/1995 P1 Annex 1

The Council (1995) offer a number of principles which it sees as underpinning the concept of preceptorship and the period of support. These are summarised as follows:

⌘ it is not an extension of a formal pre-registration programme

⌘ it does not compromise individual professional accountability which is in place at the point of registration

⌘ levels of responsibility should continue to be matched with experience

⌘ the provision of support should not affect the employment grade

⌘ support should be available for practitioners entering a new field of practice, as well as for those entering practice for the first time

⌘ practitioners returning to practice following a break of five years or more, should also be provided with similar support after completing a return to practice programme. The length of the support period may vary according to individual need

⌘ support provision should be made in all areas of practice including the private and independent sectors and for those nurse who work as Agency or Bank staff

⌘ those who are not able to find employment immediately following registration, should be provided with support on entering professional practice

The role of the preceptor

The Council (1995b) see the function of preceptorship being carried out by first level nurses, midwives or health visitors with at least twelve months of relevant experience. They may be in a full- or part-time appointment and should be willing and able to share their knowledge skills with the new entrant.

Preceptors may be identified from existing teams or from an associated area of practice. These arrangements will need to be locally determined.

Following preparation, preceptors should have achieved the following outcomes:

⌘ have sufficient knowledge of the programme that the new practitioner has followed

⌘ be able to identify the learning needs of the new practitioner

⌘ facilitate the application of theory to practice by the new practitioner

⌘ facilitate the integration of the new practitioner into the practice setting

⌘ assist in the smooth passage of the new practitioner from the role of pre-registration student to that of accountable, professional practitioner

The development of the preceptorship role, crucial to the idea of maintaining appropriate peer support, began in the pre-registration years using the mentorship vehicle. We need to document and communicate good practice and experience in both of these areas. The personal portfolio could provide an initial effective means of doing this. The Council itself:

> `...would welcome continuing contact with the professions on this issue, either to hear of other examples of policy into practice or to share its information with colleagues.'
>
> (p5 UKCC 1995b)

Clinical supervision

The discussion so far has identified professional support at two levels:

⌘ mentorship provided by suitably experienced registered nurses for pre-registration students

⌘ preceptorship provided by suitably experienced registered nurses for the newly registered professional practitioner for the first four months of professional practice

These are quite specific periods of support and should not be confused with the concept of **clinical supervision** which is now being explored to facilitate professional development and support throughout professional life.

The Vision for the Future document (Department of Health 1993) explains clinical supervision as:

> `...a term used to describe a formal process of professional support and learning which enables individual practitioners to develop knowledge and competence, assume responsibility for their own practice, and enhance consumer protection and safety of care in complex clinical situations. It is central to the

process of learning and to the expansion of the scope of practice, and should be seen as a means of encouraging self-assessment and analytical and reflective skills.'

However, much development work is currently being carried out to address issues such as those outlined by Moores (1994):

⌘ different definitions of clinical supervision

⌘ different models and systems to provide clinical supervision

⌘ local needs, facilities and resources for clinical supervision

The use of personal portfolios by professional practitioners could make a valuable contribution to this development, in addition to the seminal work that has already been done by Faugier and Butterworth (1993; 1994).

In summary, your periodic registration profile will not require information from your portfolio on your school days, personal life, leisure interests and other activities outside work. It will require evidence (which is self-verified) about your professional work experience to date, your formal continuing education achievements (both professional and academic), developments in practice, and a goal plan for your development needs. You will receive further information from the UKCC about the precise requirement when you next receive your re-registration documentation. However, there is no time like the present to get started on the material that has already been identified.

Chapter 5

Profiles for continuing professional education

In the previous chapter, there was a brief examination of the goal-setting section of your portfolio, which was closely related to the essential requirement of statutory periodic registration. We identified that an important part of the process of periodic registration is the need to submit to the UKCC a personal professional profile, which has been self-verified in the first instance. This requirement will begin to be implemented from 1 April 1998 and will be fully in place for all practitioners by the year 2001. The strategy which the UKCC will use to check that their requirements are being met has also been discussed. In this chapter, there will be a discussion of a variety of other profiles which may be required of you by both the UKCC and the appropriate National Board (depending on the part of the United Kingdom in which you are currently practising). I will use the English National Board's (ENB) Framework for Continuing Professional Education (1990) as an example in this chapter. Discussion will be developed to look, in more detail, at how the Framework relates to the UKCC statutory requirements already mentioned briefly in chapter four. In addition, there will be a consideration of new areas which will include:

- ⌘ return to practice after a career break of five years or more
- ⌘ the Higher Award (ENB)
- ⌘ the Specialist Practitioner (UKCC)
- ⌘ the Advanced Practitioner (nursing and midwifery)

UKCC profile requirements

In addition to the periodic registration regulations, discussed in chapter four, the UKCC have other specific requirements which relate to breaks in practice of five years or more. Chapter four specified what constitutes a 'break in practice' and highlights the need to record hours worked in your personal professional profile.

Statutory Return to Practice programmes will be approved by National Boards to meet the Council's requirements. If you undertake such a programme, it must be carefully documented and verified (by yourself and/or others) in your personal profile. Those parts of the programme that you undertake in the practice area must be supervised until you have completed the programme satisfactorily and have been assessed as a safe and competent practitioner in order for your registration to be renewed. This requirement will be in place from 1 April 2000 (existing legislation already requires midwives to do this).

You should be provided with appropriate written documentation of the practical, as well as the theoretical, progress that you make. If you are not, you should request it and keep it safely in your profile.

A Return to Practice programme can range from five to twenty-one days of study, in addition to appropriate supervised practice. It should be specifically tailored to your needs, which will depend upon your existing qualifications, the length of time that you have spent away from practice and your experience (including the kind of activities that you were involved in during your break). It is, therefore, important that you maintain your personal portfolio during such breaks from practice. You will then be able to produce a profile from your collection which will help your Return to Practice programme planner to identify your needs.

There are specific learning outcomes which the UKCC require you to achieve on completion of a Return to Practice programme. These include:

⌘ understanding relevant health and social policy

⌘ understanding relevant legislation, guidelines, codes of practice and policies

⌘ understanding the local and national structure and organisation of care

⌘ understanding current issues in professional education and practice

- ⌘ the use of relevant research to inform practice
- ⌘ the ability to assess, plan, implement and evaluate care
- ⌘ the ability to demonstrate communication, teaching and learning skills
- ⌘ the ability to demonstrate multi-disciplinary team working
- ⌘ the ability to demonstrate reflective practice
- ⌘ the ability to demonstrate the knowledge and skills to provide safe, competent practice

The National Boards will provide details of Return to Practice programmes, along with information about how to apply for them, nearer to the date of implementation (1 April 2000).

The ENB Framework

The Framework for Continuing Professional Education and the ENB Higher Award for Nurses, Midwives and Health Visitors are designed to help nurses practising in England fulfil the requirements of the UKCC - there are similar schemes being introduced in the other three UK countries. They began operation in April 1992 and should be considered alongside the UKCC's (1994a) requirements, discussed in the previous chapter. The requirements focus on the progression of the practitioner from:

1. Newly qualified practitioner requiring a preceptor

2. Professional practitioner

3. Specialist practitioner

4. Advanced practitioner (nursing and midwifery practice)

The ENB Framework offers an organised structure through which you can move towards different levels of practice. Until now, continuing education for nurses has been badly organised, repetitive and of dubious value. The ENB Framework offers a more coherent system which should have a much greater relevance to what you need in terms of professional/personal development and what your client needs in terms of the service you offer.

To distinguish between the UKCC proposals and the ENB Framework, it is important to acknowledge that the UKCC is responsible for the standards and levels of post-registration education and the statutory framework within which it takes place. It is, therefore, the body which endorses your legal qualifications and sets the standards. The ENB Framework is offering you the means to achieve these standards (based on the ten key areas of skill, knowledge and expertise) by a series of modular programmes which can be specially tailored to your requirements, in order for you to meet the needs of your clients. The programmes may consist of a combination of already existing ENB-approved courses, newly developed modules, qualifications awarded by other bodies (e.g. universities), credit for prior learning and modules of study from existing externally validated courses. These programmes will offer points or credits which will be collected by the practitioner towards the ENB Higher Award. The ENB will require a total of 360 credits (120 credits at levels 1, 2 and 3) as a minimum to qualify for the Higher Award. Three hundred and sixty credits (at levels 1, 2 and 3) is also the equivalent value of a three-year, full-time degree course. Further discussion of the credit system (CATS) will be included in Chapter 6. Should you wish to embark on this route, you will need to use the ENB portfolio pack to document your activities and also be indexed by the ENB.

The ENB has identified ten key characteristics to which the professional nurse should aspire as a basis for professional development. In addition, these ten characteristics define the essential areas of skills, knowledge and expertise development which are expected of the practitioner in order to qualify for the Higher Award. It would be worth keeping a copy of the ten points in the goals section of your portfolio so that you can then reflect on your own progress in achieving them. The UKCC has also stated the criteria for a specialist and an advanced practitioner.

Before we go on to discuss the accumulation of credits and how experience can be accredited, I think it might be helpful to put the ENB's ten key points and the UKCC specialist and advanced practice criteria side by side and see how they relate to each other (see Table 5.1).

	Higher Award (10 key characteristics)	**Specialist Practice**	**Advanced Practice**
1	Accountability & responsibility	Accountability & responsibility	Accountability & responsibility
2	Clinical skills with a specific client group	High level clinical skills to meet additional specialist needs	Advancing clinical practice
3	Use of research to improve care	Contributing to research & applying findings	Advancing research to enrich practice
4	Team working & building with a multi-disciplinary team	Professional leadership	Pioneering
5	Flexible & innovative approaches to care	Clinical practice development	Developing new roles
6	Use of health promotion strategies	Care & programme management	Contributing to the determination of health needs
7	Facilitating & assessing development in others	Support & supervision of colleagues	Advancing education to enrich practice

	Higher Award (*10 key characteristics*)	**Specialist Practice**	**Advanced Practice**
8	Resource management Handling information & making informed clinical decisions	Clinical nursing audit	Contribute to health policy & management
9	Quality of care Setting standards & evaluating quality	Monitor & improve standards of care	Enriching professional practice as a whole
10	Management of change Instigating, managing & evaluating clinical change	Devise new approaches to care	Adjusting the boundaries

Table 5.1: A comparison of the Higher Award (ENB) and the Specialist/Advanced Practitioner Criteria (UKCC)

Fulfilling the requirements for the Higher Award

I am sure that you will be one of many nurses asking questions such as:

> *'How far do the qualifications I have now count towards the ENB Higher Award?'*

and

> *'Does the achievement of the ENB Higher Award allow me to register as a specialist practitioner?'*

The answer to the first question depends on whether, after being indexed, you can demonstrate that you have achieved 360 credits and can submit the special ENB **Professional Portfolio** (the ENB use this term rather than the term profile) as evidence for the achievement of the ten key characteristics.

If you have completed a Project 2000 course which offers a statutory qualification, such as RGN, and a Diploma of Higher Education, you will already have acquired 240 credits (120 credits at level 1 and 120 at level 2). In addition, you will need to 'top up' with a further 120 credits at level 3. This could be achieved by completing a two-year part-time degree course. By undertaking such a course, you will probably be able to obtain evidence to confirm that you are developing some or all of the **10 Key Characteristics**. For example, most post-registration degree courses expect students to complete small research projects which relate to the students' own areas of practice. Successful completion of such a project is likely to demonstrate that you are developing in relation to numbers 1, 2,3,5,8,9 and 10 (see Table 5.1). There may be potential within the course to demonstrate other key characteristics, such as number 4 which covers team building and working, as well as multi-disciplinary team leadership. An assignment in the course, in a module of study addressing management issues, may well give you the opportunity to analyse and evaluate how you organise and lead your team. You could seek extra verification from team members and your line manager. The characteristic of facilitating and assessing development in others (number 7) can be shown through the completion of a variety of formal/informal teaching courses from

Certificate in Education, City and Guilds 730, Field Work Teacher to 'in-house' courses on teaching and assessing. Additional verification could be obtained from the staff of the College of Nursing with whom you work or from students and/or colleagues about the quality of your staff-development skills.

The relationship between the Higher Award and Specialist Practice

The ENB (1991), when developing the Higher Award, saw this as a basis for further progression.

> *'The Higher Award provides the basis for any further development of professional skills, knowledge and expertise including specialist, advanced and consultant levels of practice' (p7)*

Now that the Council's (1994c) requirements for the qualification of specialist practitioner have been unveiled, the National Boards will need to expand the Frameworks for Continuing Education to include specialist practice modules. This expansion will provide increased opportunities for those practitioners seeking either a generic or specialist Higher Award, with the added allure of registration as a specialist practitioner for the latter.

Transitional arrangements will be made to manage the integration of existing courses, the National Frameworks and the specialist programmes as they come on stream. If you are a wise practitioner, you will keep an up-to-date personal portfolio, in order to be able to take advantage of these exciting new opportunities.

Specialist practice

The Council (1994c) acknowledge that:

> *'Specialist practitioner intervention and leadership are likely to be needed in most areas of clinical practice. Patients and clients should have access to specialist care wherever nursing*

care is given. This will not require every practitioner to become a specialist.' (p4)

This statement clarifies the necessity to maintain the already existing generic Framework for those nurses who will not need or want to become specialists but still wish to progress their professional development beyond the minimum requirement of five days of study.

Specialist practitioners are expected to demonstrate:

'...higher levels of clinical decision-making and will be able to monitor and improve standards of care through supervision of practice; clinical audit; the provision of skilled professional leadership and the development of practice through research, teaching and the support of professional colleagues.' (p3, UKCC 1994c)

The Council (1994c) stipulate that programmes for specialist practice will have to be in place by the Autumn of 1998 and that these programmes will focus on four areas of study:

⌘ clinical practice
⌘ clinical practice development
⌘ care and programme management
⌘ clinical practice leadership

Areas of specialist practice other than those in the community have not been identified. This will offer flexibility and innovation at local level, particularly in terms of individual initiatives which respond to national policy, such as the reduction of the junior doctor's hours and the Scope Professional Practice (UKCC 1992). The areas of specialist practice for the community have been defined as follows:

⌘ General Practice Nursing
⌘ Community Mental Health Nursing
⌘ Community Mental Handicap Nursing
⌘ Community Children's Nursing
⌘ Public Health Nursing - Health Visiting
⌘ Occupational Health Nursing
⌘ Community Nursing in the Home - District Nursing

Figure 5.1: An Overview of Professional/Academic
Progression

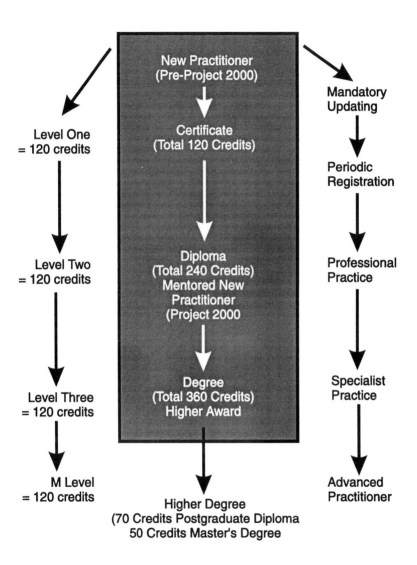

Framework for the ENB Higher Award

⌘ School Nursing

The need for maintaining your personal portfolio has already been emphasised. If you have included a specialist practice qualification in your goal setting for the future, your up-to-date portfolio will be even more vital for the following reasons:

⌘ the programme will probably be linked with a higher education accreditation system

⌘ you should be offered credit for appropriate prior learning, including learning by experience

⌘ the programme will be equally divided between theory and practice (50:50)

⌘ the modules will be at first degree level

Most programmes will be one academic year (32 weeks) full-time or the equivalent part-time. However, it should be possible for some practitioners to achieve the qualification in a shorter period of time, if claims for credit are successful. Hence the maintenance of a dynamic profile!

Transitional arrangements

Some practitioners will alrady have clinical recordable qualifications. If these courses were of at least four months duration, no further study will be required. However, further study may be needed in the following circumstances:

⌘ if the qualification is not relevant to current practice

⌘ the qualification's `shelf life' has been exceeded (usually by more than five years)

⌘ the qualification has not been consolidated by appropriate experience

Alternatively, if you have been engaged in specialist practice for at least five years, without a qualification, you could use your portfolio to produce a profile in support of an APEL (Accreditation of Prior Experiential Learning : see chapter 6) claim through an educational

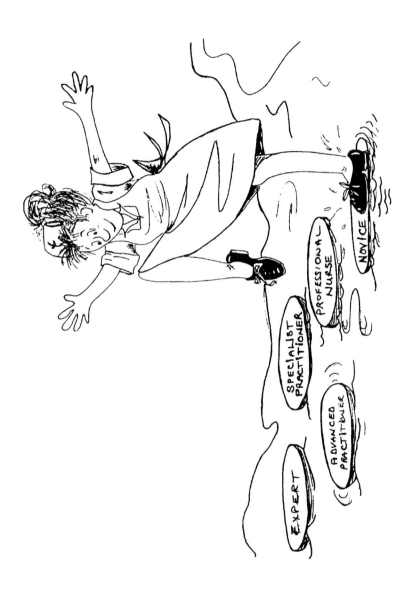

institution. This facility for claiming a whole qualification in this way may only be available for a limited period of time. The Council is still in the process of confirming these transitional arrangements. Practitioners would be well advised to maintain effective portfolios to take advantage of any new opportunities for recognition of existing expertise.

Opportunities for second-level nurses

Figure 5.1 shows how the progression might appear for both Project 2000 and non-Project 2000 practitioners, including second level nurses.

This latter point is crucial for both the career development and access to post-registration education of second level nurses. These nurses are eligible for indexing for the Higher Award including the route to a specialist practice qualification. The UKCC (1994c) specify that second level nurses should be offered a specialist programme which ensures that they:

> `...have achieved the outcomes for first level registration together with the outcomes for the specialist qualification by the completion of the programme.' (page 6)

Using this mechanism, the second level nurse should be able to use a Higher Award specialist route, not only to register as a specialist practitioner, but also to convert to first level status.

However, not all second level nurses will wish to become specialist practitioners. All frameworks for continuing education offered by the National Boards could now take the opportunity to follow the good practice of the Welsh National Board and ensure that all second level nurses can be offered a similar mechanism for conversion. This could be effected by following a generic Higher Award route and achieving the learning outcomes for first level registration at the same time.

Second-level nurses have much to gain from this more flexible framework. All qualified nurses have the opportunity to progress along the route by a variety of means, including study days, accredited experience and seminars. Educational providers are re-planning current courses, i.e. ENB certificate, attendance and competence, with a more rational modularised framework of post-registration education which is credit rated. This will considerably reduce duplication and allow greater flexibility. There will be the capacity to 'pick and mix' according to your individual needs and those of your client group. This method will considerably increase professional development opportunities for all practising nurses, both first and second level, Project 2000 or non-Project 2000. There will continue to be a mixture of ENB courses and newly validated modules of study, in addition to externally validated courses, such as part-time diploma/degree courses for some time. However, as the market demand for specialist and advanced programmes becomes clearer, a more rational approach to continuing education will emerge and opportunities for all nurses will continue to expand.

Contracts for high-quality care

The common aim of practitioners, managers and educationists is to facilitate the delivery of high standards of health to the general public. This requires that there should be a high level of co-operation and collaboration between the three groups. A major contribution towards this goal is the maintenance of an expert nursing work force which is confident, competent and compassionate. Therefore, the individual practitioner needs to negotiate agreements with:

1. The manager in relation to achieving specific developmental goals which should coincide with what the organisation is striving to provide in response to the health care needs of the general public

2. The educational establishment in order that they might facilitate the fulfilment of (1) above

The ENB (1994) offer a useful guide for purchasers and providers to utilise the Framework in relation to identifying the benchmarks that the skills and qualities of expert nurses provide. These are outlined as follows:

As a Purchaser you can use the 10 Key Characteristics to:

⌘ demonstrate the quality of the service provided by identifying the characteristics of expert practice in the work of providers

⌘ confirm the state of readiness of providers to respond to the changing needs of the community

⌘ audit the service offered by providers

⌘ monitor contracts and assess whether they are effective and efficient

As a Provider you can use the 10 Key Characteristics to:

⌘ review the skills of your staff and their ability to meet changing health care targets

⌘ make sure you have up-to-date information about the capabilities and state of readiness of your staff to set up new services or change the pattern of existing ones

⌘ make a rapid response to contract demands for new services based on informed knowledge of the skills of your staff

⌘ inform the education contracting process by making sure that education is relevant to service needs and not repetitive (p3, ENB 1994)

The learning contract between the practitioner and the educational institution is an essential pre-requisite before enrolling on a programme of study leading to the ENB Higher Award, whether this is for specialist or generic practice. Thus, four stages are involved in the process of devising an appropriate route for the individual practitioner. These stages are:

1. Review of the current stage of professional development

2. Identification of professional development need

3. Locating appropriate modules of study

4. Ongoing assessment of professional development

For the generic practitioner, all of these stages use the ten key characteristics as a basis, alongside of which learning outcomes can be checked. We could take key characteristic number 3: 'Using research to plan, implement and evaluate strategies to improve care' as an example to examine the development of a staff nurse working on a general medical ward. S/he may demonstrate, in the review process, an awareness of research in relation to managing the care of the unconscious patient. S/he may have difficulty in terms of evaluating research findings, relating relevant findings to practice, and subsequently monitoring and evaluating practice as a consequence of research-based changes in care. A programme of study could be identified to address these developmental needs. Careful assessment of professional development would be carried out. The acquisition of skills in this specific area would also contribute to the enhancement of other characteristics, i.e:

Number 5	`flexible and innovative approaches to care'`
Number 8	`handling information and making informed clinical decisions'`
Number 9	`setting standards and evaluating quality of care'`
Number 10	`instigating, managing and evaluating clinical change'`

For this reason, the ten key points should not be viewed in isolation but rather as an integrated whole when planning professional development programmes.

The same processes will apply for the practitioner who wishes to embark on a specialist practice route. Table 5.1 illustrates the expanded role required for specialist practice. Some practitioners who have already indexed for the Higher Award may need to make only minor adjustments to their study route in order to convert to a specialist practitioner programme. Using the earlier example of the staff nurse working on the medical ward, s/he may be able to demonstrate a high level of clinical skill in diabetic care which has been supported by appropriate theoretical study at level 3. S/he may also have taken a significant part in a clinical audit of urinalysis documentation as part of routine admission assessments across ten wards in his/her hospital. As a consequence of this work, s/he may have been able to devise new approaches to care and offer support/supervision of colleagues. S/he needs further development in relation to leadership skills. A further module of study has been identified to address this and clinical supervision to assess his/her progress has been offered.

Clearly, there is a requirement here for a contract or agreement between the educational and service providers who are responding to the requirements of the purchasing health authority. The health authority has the overall responsibility for purchasing the right level and quality of health care. In our multiple roles as professional practitioners, trainees, users of health care services and tax payers, we are both purchasers and providers of this essential facility. We should not need better motivation than this in getting our contracts right.

Advanced practice

Figure 5.1 demonstrates the progression of the post-registration of nurses in the following stages:

1. Professional practice supported by preceptor for approximately four months

2. Professional practice, which immediately follows the support stage, when consolidation and further development of skills takes place. It is likely that most practitioners will remain in this category, which has a minimum requirement of five days updating every three years, with the option of indexing for a generic Higher Award

3. Specialist practice follows a period of additional specific education within a clearly defined area of practice

4. Advanced practice can develop from specialist practice or develop alongside it, so that there is some overlap between the two. The advanced practitioner is able to lead effectively and has a high level of analytical ability. The range of skills is wide and embraces direct care, education, management and research

The earlier deliberations of the UKCC (1990) had indicated the possibility of a recorded qualification for advanced practice. This, however, has now been postponed for the time being on the grounds that the Council (1995) do not wish to restrict innovation or stifle progress in the development of this new concept. Council expect practitioners who are acquiring advanced skills to be educated to higher degree level. A good example of this kind of preparation is the Postgraduate Diploma/MSc in Advanced Nursing Practice currently being offered by the University of Central England in Birmingham. Students on this programme are beginning to make a significant contribution to our understanding of advanced practice in the UK (Brown 1995; Paniagua 1995). They have also taken to heart the UKCC's (1995) valuable advice in taking the opportunity:

> *'...to demonstrate, through your professional profile, that you have achieved a level of practice and professional knowledge that equates with the concept of advanced practice. This will help to develop your career, and your examples of good practice will also assist the UKCC in its development work in this area' (Fact Sheet 7).*

While the UKCC do not see advanced practice as an extra layer of practice in addition to specialist practice, they are acknowledging that some practitioners will have the potential to develop further and should not be restricted from so doing by the framework that is currently in place.

Advanced practice for both nurses and midwives is defined by Council (1995) as being concerned with:

- ⌘ Adjusting the boundaries for the development of future practice
- ⌘ Pioneering and developing new roles which are responsive to changing needs
- ⌘ Advancing clinical practice, research and education to enrich professional practice as a whole
- ⌘ Contributing to health policy and management and the determination of health needs
- ⌘ Continuing the development of the professions in the interest of patients, clients and health services

It is asserted that by advancing practice in this way, there will be:

- ⌘ Innovations in practice
- ⌘ An increase in research and research-based practice
- ⌘ The provision of expert professionals who will have a consultancy role
- ⌘ High level professional leadership
- ⌘ Increased political and professional influence in respect of the development of maternity/nursing/health services
- ⌘ Expert resources, for example education, supervision and management (Fact Sheet 7, UKCC 1995).

This vision, on the part of the Council, offers practitioners exciting possibilities for developments in client care with which to go forward into the twenty-first century.

Chapter 6

Putting your CATS among the profiles

Introduction

The previous chapter introduced the idea that new qualifications, such as the specialist practitioner (UKCC) and the Higher Award (ENB) could be achieved by the accumulation of credits. This means that both the achievements of the past and the things that you want to do in the future may be given an academic value in terms of the level and amount of learning that you have now and will achieve in the future.

During the 1970s, I began studying for an Open University degree in my own time. When I was two-thirds of the way through the work, I tried to gain access to a conventional university to complete my final year in full-time study. I think I approached virtually every university in England but not one of them had a procedure which enabled them to acknowledge the learning that I had already accomplished. I am really quite envious of the new system of accreditation which is available to you now but was not in existence when I needed it.

Accreditation of learning can be done by:

1. A formal **Credit Accumulation and Transfer System** in which credits are accumulated from existing recordable qualifications and/or by successfully completing formal courses of study, which have a specific credit value at a particular level, e.g. a Diploma in Professional Studies in Nursing (120 credits at level 2)

2. **Assessment/Accreditation of Prior Learning** (APL). This can include everything that you have ever learned by whatever method and can range from your everyday experiences to your formal qualifications.

3. **Assessment/Accreditation of Prior Experiential Learning** (APEL). This applies to anything that you have learned by experience. It usually excludes learning which is semi-formally or formally assessed by tests, projects, practicals, assessments, examinations etc.

The Credit Accumulation System will be discussed first and then the Assessment of Prior Learning. Our discussions should help you to use your personal portfolio as a database to produce profiles that utilise the two systems. This will both support your professional development, as well as enable you to make viable claims for learning already achieved. You may then choose whether or not you wish to use this accreditation in order to obtain a specific qualification.

Credit accumulation and transfer

The CATS system was introduced in the mid-1980s by the Council for National Academic Awards (CNAA), the body which validated awards, such as degrees in higher education institutions, e.g. polytechnics. The aim of the CAT scheme was to provide additional opportunities for you as an individual by:

⌘ giving credit for what you have already learned

⌘ enabling you to collect this credit towards an academic award

⌘ enabling you to put together units of study appropriate to your needs (CNAA 1986)

CATS incorporates the possibility of:

⌘ CREDIT EXEMPTION—your previous learning may allow you to be exempted from a particular part of a course

⌘ CREDIT TRANSFER—enables you to transfer the credits that you have already acquired between courses, either inside or across institutional boundaries thus allowing flexibility

⌘ CREDIT ACCUMULATION—you can collect credits from a range of learning experiences and use them towards obtaining a qualification

For credit to be given, learning must be assessed to ensure that it has taken place at the appropriate level. Table 6.1 illustrates how such levels relate to nursing qualifications and the number of credits required for each level. Looking at your own qualifications and experience along side the ENB's ten key characteristics should help you to make an initial judgement about how far you have progressed towards fulfilling the requirements for the Higher Award. Appendix 1 contains a specimen CV for a fictitious nurse called Bernice Hamilton. Bernice was able to do a pre-registration course (Registered Mental Nurse) to diploma level because the course was validated by both the ENB and an institution of higher education (conjoint validation). By doing this, she has acquired 120 credits at levels 1 and 2 (240 credits in all). Since qualifying, she has gained a further 60 credits at level 3 for a new conjointly validated modularised course on adult behavioural psychotherapy (consisting of four modules of study worth fifteen credits each). The modules focused on the theory and practice of psychotherapy, ethico/legal issues and the management of change.

To qualify for the Higher Award she will need to:

1.   Acknowledge that she still needs a further 60 credits at level 3

2.   Review her achievements and expertise in relation to the ten key characteristics

3.   Index with the ENB for the Higher Award and obtain the ENB Personal Portfolio pack

4.   Identify the learning outcomes which she still needs to achieve

5.   Agree to a contract with both the educational institution and her managers so that the learning opportunities which she requires can be both provided for her and used by her

6.   Achieve the learning outcomes which must be assessed in order to gain the Higher Award

Table 6.1: The Credit Accumulation and Transfer System (CATS)

LEVEL 1	120 credits	= the equivalent of the standard of study undertaken at certificate level or in the first year of a degree course
	(A post-1985 first level qualification i.e. RGN = minimum 60 level 1 credits)	
LEVEL 2	120 credits	= the equivalent of the standard of study undertaken at diploma level or in the second year of a degree course
	(A post-1982 London University Diploma in Nursing = 60 credits at level 1 and 120 credits at level 2)	
LEVEL 3	120 credits	= the equivalent of the standard of study undertaken in the third year of a degree course
	(A two-year, part-time, post-registration BSc (Hons) Nursing Studies = 120 credits at level 3)	
TOTAL	360 credits	= Degree with honours
LEVEL M	120 credits	= the equivalent of the standard of study undertaken for a post-graduate diploma/master's degree
1 credit	= equivalent of approximately 8 hours of study, not necesarily college-based	
1 experientia lcredit (APEL)	= equivalent of approximately 16 hours of practice	

Assessment of prior learning including experiential

Bernice could acquire the final 60 level 3 credits by APEL (Assessment of Prior Experiential Learning). It is permissible to acquire up to fifty per cent of credits for one level by this method but it must be assessed. Prior experiential learning has been defined by the Further Education Unit (1983) as:

> '*...the knowledge and skills acquired through life and work experience and study which are not formally attested through any educational or professional certification.*'

It is Bernice's responsibility to make a claim for prior learning which fulfils the requirements of the ten key characteristics and can be equated with a minimum of 60 credits at level 3. For example, Bernice, along with her educational adviser, may agree that further evidence is required to support the achievement of the following key characteristics:

1. Clinical expertise with a specific client group;

2. Flexible and innovative approaches to care; and

3. Handling information and making informed clinical decisions.

Bernice could then complete these requirements by passing through the following stages to develop her evidence of prior learning in readiness for assessment.

Stages in making a claim

Stage 1

She could consider her personal, professional and study experiences and identify areas or activities when learning occurred which contributed to the three specified key characteristics:

1. Personal experiences – consider how she is treated as an individual in a family

2. Professional experiences – strategies that she uses both personally and as a team leader to emphasise the patient's individuality

3. Study experiences – study days/seminars/conferences attended which have focused on primary nursing. Articles read and private study

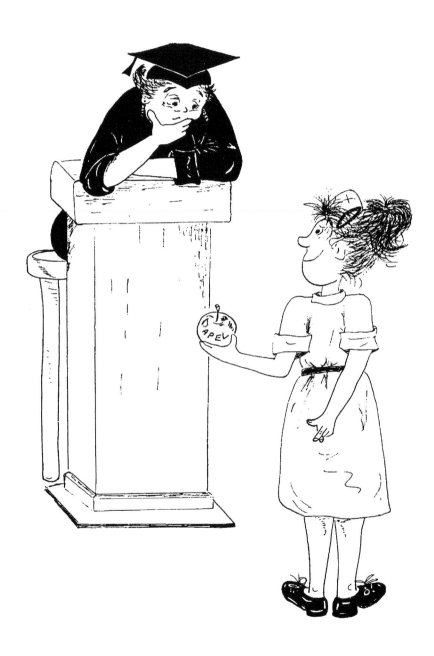

Stage 2

Bernice could write down what she learned from these experiences in the form of learning outcomes, e.g:

> *'I can understand the need for everyone, both carers and cared for, to express their individuality.'*

> *'I can critically evaluate the relevant literature in relation to primary nursing as a means of individualising care.'*

> *'I can apply theory to practice in relation to care delivery.'*

> *'I can critically evaluate care that is given by myself and others.'*

Stage 3

She could collect evidence to support the claims made for learning. An important dimension of this is how well Bernice performs as a professional practitioner. The evidence of this may be provided in a variety of ways by both Bernice and others. Some conclusions about the quality of practice on the ward might be drawn from a survey of patients' satisfaction, progress and support of learners and evidence of innovation. The operation of an individual performance review system and observation of Bernice in action will also contribute to a knowledge about her professional practice.

Bernice could provide a written account of how she has introduced and evaluated primary nursing in her ward, possibly including an analysis of the suitability of this approach to care for the particular client group with which she is working. She may further develop her account to discuss the notion of primary nursing acting as a vehicle for sensitive, informed clinical decision-making. The account should include evidence of critical use of the literature. Bernice may also have attended conferences and seminars.

Stage 4

At this stage, the experiences, learning outcomes and evidence are put together to form a complete entry in Bernice's profile to support her application. The application is then assessed by a named person for the institution carrying out the Assessment of Prior Experiential Learning. The assessor will be judging whether the learning outcomes, which were identified in relation to the key characteristics, were achieved. The assessment will be documented in Section Three of the ENB Professional Portfolio folder.

Learning outcomes

Stage 2 of the APEL process is very important in terms of identifying what has been learned (learning outcomes). The clarity with which learning outcomes are expressed can be enhanced by the use of words which describe exactly what you have learned and what you can do as a result of this learning. For example:

⌘ Understand legal issues in relation to care of the mentally ill. Demonstrate how this understanding is applied to practice.

⌘ Demonstrate and apply knowledge of relevant life sciences (such as sociology/biology) to the care of the mentally ill

⌘ Promote team building and, in so doing, create and utilise a common philosophy of care

Because Bernice needs to provide evidence of prior learning at level 3 (which is similar to that level of learning achieved during the final year of a degree course) particular attention will be paid to her demonstration of higher level skills. These higher level skills are necessary to handle areas of knowledge which become increasingly complicated. Educationists sometimes use a framework developed by Steinaker and Bell (1979) to identify different levels of learning. Lower levels of learning are depicted by the ability to define and describe, while higher levels are those that demonstrate an advanced level of mastery in relation to deductive reasoning skills, critical analysis, synthesis and creative thought. The developing skill base is a balanced mixture of having an appropriate level of knowledge which is reflected in what you do and the attitudes which you convey. Knowledge can be acquired by being exposed (or by actively seeking exposure) to an everyday experience, exploring and reflecting on the experience, trying out what you have learned from it, and using your new awareness to influence other people and situations.

For example, take the simple everyday task of Bernice carrying out a bed bath. Bernice's assessor could use the above criteria to observe Bernice as she demonstrates a high level of expertise in areas which include:

1. Manual dexterity in handling the patient and the equipment

2. Organisational skills in preparing the setting

3. Sensitivity to the maintenance of privacy

4. Verbal and non-verbal communication skills

5. Observation and problem identification

6. Negotiation with client and colleagues

7. Positive role model to the ward team

8. Organisational features of primary nursing

9. Critical analysis and reflection on care giving

Our expectations of a student in training would be very different, particularly if it was her/his first involvement in such a procedure. In this case, s/he would be experiencing the very low level of Steinaker and Bell's cycle (1979), usually defined as exposure. S/he would be anxious about this new experience and would have limited knowledge and experience on which to draw. In Bernice's case, the assessor would take on the role of a critic. In the case of the new learner, the teacher would be a facilitator and motivator.

Using Bernice as an example has, I hope, helped to highlight how a more recently qualified nurse might progress through the ENB framework and use it to 'top up' existing qualifications. The example has focused on APEL. Bernice could equally have chosen to have obtained the 60 credits by successfully completing an accredited, modularised level 3 course. The course would be selected to match the outstanding criteria that Bernice was expected to meet in relation to the ten key characteristics. Similar principles can still be applied for nurses who have been qualified rather longer.

Most nurses should be able to justify a credit rating of 120 credits at level 1. This will be easier for those of you who qualified after 1985 because, at that time, the ENB and CNAA mutually agreed the credit rating for registration and some post-registration qualifications. For example, the Health Visitors' Certificate attracted 110 credits at level 1 and 30 credits at level 2. It is highly likely that someone with this kind of profile could provide enough evidence using APEL to gain the remaining ten credits at level 1 and at the same time undertake a 'top up' course to diploma level to complete the level 2 work. S/he would then need to consider plans for obtaining 120 credits at level 3. This could be achieved 'in one fell swoop' by taking a two-year part-time post-registration degree in nursing or health studies. Alternatively, a package of modularised, conjointly validated courses is available which can be taken on a 'pick and mix' basis, according to specific individual needs in terms of attendance mode, content, pace and time span. This offers greater flexibility and is a very attractive proposition.

A nurse who qualified pre-1985 will have to make a case through the APL system, in terms of his/her registration qualifications and other formal qualifications, as well as assessing prior experiential learning. A balance of 50/50 for each level is acceptable in relation to formal qualifications and learning from experience. Most nurses who qualified pre-1985 should be able to justify 60 credits at level 1 for formal qualifications and 60 credits on APEL. Additionally, some qualifications, such as registration as a clinical teacher, will attract some credit exemption from level 2 work. Your own credit rating will be something that is individual to you and should be judged as such. Everyone's career is slightly different, as are the learning outcomes that you have achieved.

The experienced nurses who present to me as candidates for the post-registration diploma and degree (levels 2 and 3) courses bring rich and varied professional profiles for assessment. Here are some examples:

> **Mrs C** *was a clinical nurse specialist in wound care. She had previously qualified as a clinical teacher and had completed ENB 870 on research. She was able to present a great deal of evidence of innovation and learning in relation to her specialist practice. She was keen to gain admission to level 3 study in order to achieve an honours degree. Following successful completion of a degree, it was her intention to*

undertake a taught masters' programme. She was awarded 120 credits at both levels 1 and 2 for prior learning.

Mr S *was a very experienced nurse working in a coronary care unit. He had first qualified as a second level nurse and had gone on to qualify as a first level nurse. His profile showed that he had far in excess of the required 120 credits at level 1. These were mostly obtained by the completion of ENB certificate, attendance or competence-based courses. He needed to establish whether his progression could be accredited at level 2. On the basis of completing the APL exercise and some additional set project work, it was possible to award him 90 credits at level 2. In practical terms, this meant that he was able to gain admission to the second year of the Diploma course. Out of the four units of study offered in that year, he was only required to do two (15 credits each), whereby he gained the required 30 credits to complete his level 2 work. He was then able to progress into level 3. He decided to complete this by undertaking the part-time, two-year honours degree. Had the ENB Higher Award been available, he may have opted to do several level 3 modules of study (to achieve 120 level 3 credits) to qualify for the Higher Award. This award is the equivalent of degree-level study.*

In summary, assessment and accreditation of prior learning (APL) can include learning from experience (APEL) as well as more formal certificated learning. When making your claim, you must provide evidence (preferably verified) about what you have learned. The person who is assessing your claim will be undertaking three tasks:

1. Establishing that learning has taken place

2. Deciding the level of the learning (1, 2 or 3)

3. Deciding the amount of credit to be awarded

At the end of the day, the aim is to make sure that you are capable of study and learning at that level and that you and the service will benefit.

This chapter has highlighted the need for skilled and knowledgeable educational advisers and assessors/verifiers. This will require an intensive and focused programme of preparation by nurse educators and others if we are to ensure that the APL approach is workable and fair.

Developing a comprehensive personal portfolio, from which a variety of profiles can be created for use in CATS and APEL, will be invaluable for your continuing professional development. You will be able to use the material to substantiate claims for such things as the ENB Higher Award, the UKCC Specialist Practitioner registration, admission to courses with advanced standing, credit exemption and periodic registration. Your efficiency in handling individual performance-review procedures will also be enhanced, so I'll leave you now to get on with putting your CATS among your profiles!

Chapter 7

An evaluation of a selection of profile packages

Introduction

Ellis (1992), in a letter to the Nursing Times, lamented about the confusion which seems to reign in relation to the different profile packs being marketed at a price by various professional bodies. She argues that nurses should be made aware of the criteria which need to be met in completing a profile for a particular purpose. However, she was alarmed that nurses might be expected to complete several profiles:

> '...surely the vital element is encouraging all practitioners to reflect as they find it easiest? It is then the job of an accreditation officer to examine each individual profile to ascertain what can be credited and at what level. It could otherwise soon be the case that a practitioner may have to possess many different profiles: her/his own, one for the ENB and one for the UKCC, one for each higher education institution s/he is applying to, and so on'

The ENB Professional Portfolio

I have endeavoured to demonstrate that flexibility is the key to managing your personal portfolio and the profiles you draw from it. A flexible approach should enable you to overcome the difficulties which Ellis (1992) anticipates. However, you may be obliged to purchase a particular profile pack if you wish to become eligible for a specific award. For example, the ENB Professional Portfolio pack is an essential element in the indexing process for the Higher Award. If you do buy the pack, you could utilise it in a broader way, i.e. you may collect additional material that could be used for other purposes, such as access to a course with advanced standing or to organise your own documentation for periodic registration. There are internal pockets inside the covers to enable you to do this.

The inside cover of the portfolio binder contains a series of useful summary cards which provide an explanatory synopsis of important areas. These are as follows:

1.   10 Key Characteristics

2.   Higher Award Learning Outcomes

3.   ENB Professional Portfolio

4.   Credit Accumulation and Transfer

5.   Pathways through the Framework

The portfolio itself is very comprehensive and contains the following sections:

1.   Qualifications and experience to date

2.   Present post

3.   Continuing professional education

4.   Becoming a reflective practitioner

5.   Summary of learning achievements

6.   General information

If you have followed the suggestions in this book, you will already have summarised a great deal of this information for your extended *curriculum vitae.*

Each of the above sections has a series of blank pages containing well organised headings. For example, the first section **'Qualifications and Experience to Date'** has clearly defined areas for professional education:

1.   Professional Registrable Qualifications:

   a)   First qualification

b)   Subsequent qualifications

2.   Recordable qualifications, e.g. National Board Certificate Courses

3   Other professional qualifications, e.g. Diploma in Nursing

4.   Professional employment record

5.   Credits towards the Higher Award

6.   Participation in continuing education

7.   Other experiences or activities

Each entry is divided into spaces for the name of the qualification and the place and date it was obtained.

This particular pack would be helpful to most nurses, whether or not they were contemplating the completion of the Higher Award. Two minor criticisms concern the overlap between professional and higher education, already discussed in Chapter 3, and the inclusion of potentially sensitive material in what, ostensibly, becomes a public document if the Higher Award is completed. The designated sections for professional and higher education make no reference to situations where a nurse may have a qualification which could go into either category. For example, a Certificate in Education may have been obtained in order for a nurse to register as a tutor. In this case, it would perhaps be helpful to record the certificate in the Higher Education section and the Registered Nurse Tutor qualification in the Professional Education section, with cross referencing.

My second reservation concerns the invitation to make statements about yourself in an 'Additional Information' section at the end of the 'qualifications and experience to date' entries. This includes information about your personality, your attributes, your hopes for the future and your performance in your current post. These are important aspects of your life on which to reflect. However, you may like to select statements which you are happy to make public and keep other more personal insights about your strengths and weaknesses as a private *aide memoire*.

The pack also offers useful advice about how to manage the contents over time. For example, it is suggested that, when you change your employment, you could summarise the section on your outgoing post and add this information to your previous employment record, before starting a fresh entry for your new job. The section also contains helpful guidelines on relating your current post to the ten key characteristics, the ENB Higher Award and your continuing education programme. The underlying emphasis is to encourage you to reflect on what you have done in the past, what you are doing now and your plans for the future.

This package has undergone a recent update (February 1995) with the adition of a `How to use' guidance booklet.

The Nursing Times Profile Pack

The Nursing Times Profile Pack is similar to the ENB Professional Portfolio in that it facilitates the documentation of your professional development and education. In addition, it acknowledges that some of your profile will be essentially private and not for public view. The pack has a structure similar to an individualised learning package which encourages you to engage in, and reflect on, self-directed activities. An example is Section 3, which is called 'Values, Attitudes and Beliefs.' Such a section is helpful because nurses sometimes find it difficult to articulate what are often seen as rather abstract ideas about their own personal philosophies and how they relate to professional practice.

The first part of the profile is constructed to help you review your current situation. It contains several activities, including a reflective diary and covers:

The Review Section	
Your Life and Times	Skills Inventory
Values, Attitudes and Beliefs	Focus on Achievement
Your Professional Life	Review Summary
What Kind of Learner are You?	Setting Goals

You are advised as to which parts could be included in the 'Professional Record' and which parts might be considered a private record.

The next section of the profile is the Professional Record which can be used for public consumption and contains the following more orthodox sections:

- ⌘ Biographical details
- ⌘ Education and training
- ⌘ Employment history
- ⌘ Professional development records
- ⌘ Additional information

The emphasis of the structure of this profile pack encourages you to think carefully about both your personal and professional life. It also contains a handy supply of master record sheets to photocopy.

The British Journal of Nursing Professional Portfolio for Nurses

The BJN portfolio pack offers a comprehensive set of sections covering:

⌘ Education	⌘ Teaching
⌘ Employment	⌘ Publications
⌘ Research	⌘ Other Activities

Each section is accompanied by appropriate information and blank documentation forms which can be photocopied. Despite the comprehensiveness of this pack, it is likely that it will have limited appeal, as the majority of nurses will have rather different components in their career profiles, particularly in relation to research, publications and teaching. This publication would have been enhanced by some in-built flexibility and the inclusion of sections on the documentation of clinical practice, in addition to a section on the private/personal experiences and reflective aspirations of the practitioner.

Midirs (Midwives Information and Resource Service) Midwifery Portfolio

This portfolio for midwives is contained in an A4 ring binder and has the following parts:

- ⌘ Introduction
- ⌘ Personal details
- ⌘ General Education, Skills and Development
- ⌘ Professional Education, Skills and Development
- ⌘ Employment History

It acknowledges the importance of non-professional education, skills and experience, and provides appropriate proforma. Plastic wallets are included in which to store certificates etc. This compilation is pleasing in that it addresses both personal and professional growth. It is flexible enough to be used by midwives (or other health care professionals for that matter) operating at a variety of levels.

The packs that I have described are useful for beginning the collection of your documentation. However, try not to become too rigid, both in how you organise your material and in terms of the things that you choose to collect. Bear in mind our earlier discussions about the creation of your personal portfolio. This could contain a variety of materials which may not be suitable for every profile that you produce.

The Welsh National Board Professional Profile

Each of the National Boards has its own approach to the framework for continuing education. While there are many similarities, there are also some differences. For example, the Welsh National Board (WNB) has produced a small, pocket-sized Professional Profile folder which is similar to a personal organiser. If you prefer something more portable as part of your portfolio collection, this could be it. Although the contents and layout conform to the WNB's framework, it could easily be adapted for use in England, Scotland or Northern Ireland. The pack contains the following sections:

- ⌘ Experience to date – including both jobs and qualifications
- ⌘ WNB Certificate and Diploma in Professional Practice (WNB Framework)
- ⌘ Professional and academic qualifications (gained after starting the Profile)
- ⌘ Becoming a reflective practitioner: using critical incidents
- ⌘ Development and performance review
- ⌘ Summary information
- ⌘ General information

This mini-file maintains the basic principles of profile keeping in an economical size which is appealing. It encourages reflection, good record keeping and professional development.

The Royal College of Nursing Professional Portfolio

The publishing arm of the Royal College of Nursing (Scutari) have also produced a personal organiser-type Professional Portfolio. This includes a diary, year planner and information pages, plus guides on topics such as:

- ⌘ the health service
- ⌘ writing a CV
- ⌘ UKCC Code of Conduct
- ⌘ getting the job you want
- ⌘ useful addresses
- ⌘ using libraries
- ⌘ further and continuing education
- ⌘ doing literature searches
- ⌘ education
- ⌘ coping with stress
- ⌘ clinical grading
- ⌘ speaking and writing effectively

- ⌘ nursing models
- ⌘ drug administration
- ⌘ chairing meetings
- ⌘ clinical information
- ⌘ ward teaching
- ⌘ PREP

Comment

As the frameworks for continuing education get underway across the United Kingdom, the number of portfolio and profile packs available for purchase will increase. I hope this book will enable you to be a discerning purchaser and help you to acquire the package that fits both your personal and professional needs. There is no doubt that life will be so much easier with your own personal portfolio.

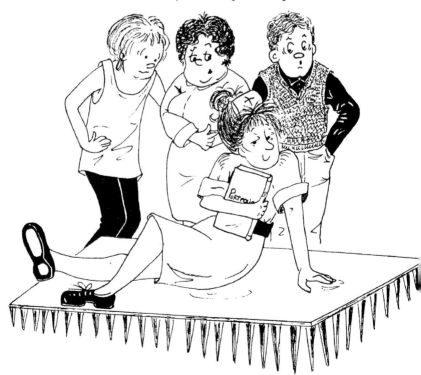

Appendix 1

Specimen *Curriculum Vitae*

Surname: HAMILTON **Age**: 28 years

Maiden Name: n/a

Forenames: Bernice Eleanor **Date of Birth**: 5 August 1966

Title: Ms **Marital Status**: Single

Address: 32 Lower St, Brindleford

Six Oaks, SO6 3LS

Telephone No Work: 01 560 127631 X 45

Home: 01 560 357290

Present Post: Junior Sister

Grade:

Present Employer: Brindleford Hospital Trust

PIN Number (UKCC):

Number and Ages of Dependants: n/a

Current Salary/Scale:

Nationality:

General Education

1977-1984   St Cecilia's Collegiate School, Six Oaks, Kent

GCSEs – 6 subjects

English Language (B)

Biology (A), Mathematics (C)

Geography (C), French (C)

Chemistry (C)

A Levels – 1 subject

Biology (C)

Higher Education

1985-1988   Mid-England College of Higher Education
Birminster, Warwicks
Diploma in Higher Education

Professional Education

1985-1988   Mid-England College of Nursing
Birminster, Warwicks
Registered Mental Nurse (UKCC)

1994   Princess Mary College of Nursing
Southmere, Hants.
Adult Behavioural Psychotherapy Course
(60 credits at level 3)

Current Post

Junior Sister, Sedgwick Clinic, Southwood – from January 1995

Role includes: acting up in the absence of the Senior Sister; mentoring, teaching and assessing learner nurses; acting as primary nurse for small case load of mixed dependency clients; evaluating the operation of primary nursing; research liaison with multi-disciplinary team in relation to current research findings.

Previous Nursing Employment

1988-1994   Rolfe Clinic Assessment Unit, Armswood, West Midlands
Staff Nurse

Non-nursing Employment

1984   Glover's Chemist, Six Oaks, Kent
Shop Assistant

Voluntary Work

1981-1985   Six Oaks Free Wheelers Club for Physically/ Mentally Handicapped Adolescents
Helper–particularly on trips and holidays

1984-1985   Six Oaks Methodist Church Youth Club
Organiser of speakers, activities, etc.

Leisure Activities

Tennis, reading, craftwork, cinema and theatre

Other Information

Currently undertaking a counselling course in preparation for work with the Samaritans. Applied to join an Open Learning programme in the Autumn

Referees

Mrs C J Talbot	Dr K N Saunders
Director of Patient Services	Clinical Psychologist
Sedgwick Clinic	Rolfe Clinic Assessment Unit
Southwood	Rolfe Clinic
Six Oaks	Armswood
Kent	West Midlands
Tel. No.	Tel. No.

Appendix 2

UKCC PIN Instructions

Ms B E Hamilton UKCC
32 Lower Street
Brindleford
Six Oaks
SO6 3LS

 PIN 10A......

Dear Colleague

I am pleased to attach your receipt card. Would you please read the information and instructions below and sign the card **immediately.**

1. This receipt card is evidence that the UKCC has received your registration fee and that you have effective registration. It ensures your right to practice on the appropriate part(s) of the Register of the UKCC until the last day of the month shown on the face of the card, unless otherwise advised earlier by the UKCC, its officers or Agents.

2. The card should enable your employer, or prospective employer, to confirm the status of your registration and should be available to them on request.

3. At not less than 45 days before the expiry date shown on your card, a renewal application will be sent to you at the address held against your name at that time.

4. You should notify the UKCC whenever you change the address to which you wish the UKCC to write when communicating with you.

5.   If the card should be lost then you are requested to inform the UKCC at once. This will assist the Council in fulfilling its role to protect the public from persons who falsely claim to be qualified practitioners.

6.   Please make a note of your Professional Identification Number (PIN), and use it on all communications with this Council.

If you have any comments or questions regarding this card, the Registration Department would be pleased to assist you.

Yours sincerely

Registrar and
Chief Executive

UNITED KINGDOM CENTRAL COUNCIL
FOR NURSING, MIDWIFERY AND HEALTH VISITING
23, Portland Place, London, W1N 3AF

Glossary

Accreditation/Assessment of Prior Experiential Learning (APEL)

⌘ Acknowledging any learning from previous experience

Accreditation/Assessment of Prior Learning (APL)

⌘ Taking into account everything that you have previously learned (formally, semi-formally, informally) which may be certificated or experiential

Advanced Practitioner

⌘ A specialist who has, among other things, leadership skills and a high level of analytical ability, and who is able to demonstrate innovation and creativity

Advanced Standing

⌘ Admission to a level of a programme of study at a later stage than a student with the minimum entry requirements

Clinical Supervision

⌘ A formal process of professional support and learning which enables individual practitioners to develop knowledge and competence, assume responsibility for their own practice and enhance consumer protection and safety of care in complex clinical situations

Competence

⌘ The ability to carry out a specific activity to an identified standard

Conjoint Validation

⌘ When a course is validated by two or more validating bodies, e.g. ENB and a university

Credit Accumulation System

⌘ In which students progress towards an award by accumulation of credits assigned to modules of study

Credit Exemption

⌘ Previous learning may allow a student exemption from a particular part of a course or module of study

Credit Transfer

⌘ One institution or course recognises and accepts credits obtained elsewhere both internally or externally to the institution

Curriculum Vitae (CV)

⌘ An outline of a person's educational and professional history

Learning Contract

⌘ A plan of action which is mutually agreed between a student and a teacher. It usually includes the assessment of prior learning; the learning outcomes which need to be achieved; the means by which these shall be achieved and the way in which learning will be assessed

Level

⌘ Modules of study may be offered at levels 1, 2 and 3. These normally correspond to undergraduate studies at Certificate, Diploma and Degree level. Postgraduate study is usually designated as M level

Mandatory

⌘ An obligatory requirement made by an authoritative body

Modularised Course

⌘ In which students progress towards an award by accumulation of credits assigned to blocks of study

Non-recordable Qualifications

⌘ Qualifications which are not recorded on the Register, e.g. ENB courses, in-house courses, City and Guilds 730

Periodic Registration

⌘ A legal requirement to register every three years with the UKCC in order to continue in practice

Personal Portfolio

⌘ A privat collection of evidence which demonstrates learning and application to professional practice

Personal Profile

⌘ Selected evidence from the portfolio which demonstrates learning for a specific purpose

Preceptor

⌘ An experienced qualified nurse who provides support for the newly qualified practitioner who is entering professional practice

PREPP

⌘ Post-Registration Education and Practice Project

Prior Experiential Learning

⌘ Knowledge, skills and attitudes acquired through life experience not formally accredited.

Professional Practice

⌘ Immediately following the support stage when skills are consolidated

Recordable Qualifications

⌘ Qualifications which are recorded by the UKCC on any part of the Register and which constitute a statutory requirement for practice, e.g. RGN, RMN, RMNH

Specialist Practice

⌘ This follows a period of specific post-registration education within a clearly defined area of practice

Statutory

⌘ A legal requirement

Verification

⌘ Evidence from self or others which confirms that learning has taken place

Acronym List

APEL	Accreditation/Assessment of Prior Experiential Learning
APL	Accreditation/Assessment of Prior Learning
CATS	Credit Accumulation and Transfer System
CV	*Curriculum Vitae*
DPSN	Diploma in Professional Studies in Nursing
ENB	English National Board
GCSE	General Certificate of Secondary Education
PIN	Professional Identification Number
PREP	Post-Registration Education and Practice
PREPP	Post-Registration Education and Practice Project
RGN	Registered General Nurse
RNMH	Registered Nurse Mental Handicap
RM	Registered Midwife
UKCC	United Kingdom Central Council for Nursing, Midwifery and Health Visiting
WNB	Welsh National Board

Bibliography

Anon (1991). PREP profile to be discussed this week, *Nurs Stand*, **6**(6), 5

Brown R A (1989). *Individualised Care: The Role of the Ward Sister*, Scutari Publications, Harrow

Brown R A (1991). The Age of Unreason and the Charge Nurse, *Nurs Stand*, **5**, 20

Brown R A (1995). Education for specialist and advanced practice, *Br J Nurs*, **4**:5

Butterworth T and Faugier J eds (1992). Clinical Supervision and Mentorship in Nursing, Chapman & Hall, London

Corfield R (1990). *Preparing Your Own CV*, Kogan Page, London

Crossland D (1991). *Assessment of Prior Learning and Achievement*, National Institute of Continuing Education

CNAA (1986). *The Credit Accumulation and Transfer System, Publication* 1a/46, CNAA, May

Department of Health (1993). A Vision for the Future, The Nursing, Midwifery and Health Visiting Contribution to Health and Health Care

Ellis J (1992). Profile for Achievement, *Nursing Times*, **88**(1)

English National Board (1991). *Professional Portfolio*, London: ENB

English National Board (1994). *Reframing the Framework. A Manager's Perspective*, London: ENB 1994

Faugier J and Butterworth C A (1993). Position paper on clinical supervision, Manchester University

FEU (1983). *Further Educational Curriculum Opportunity - a map of experiential learning in entry requirements to higher and further education award-bearing courses*, FEU, May

Hand D (1991). PREP, *Nursing Standard*, **5**(44)

Houle C O (1980). *Continuing Learning in the Professions*, Jossey-Bass, San Francisco

McSweeney P (1991). The Collapse of the Conventional Career, *Nursing Times,* **87**(31)

Moores Y (1994). CNO Professional Letter 94 (5), Department of Health, London

Nursing Times (1993), *The Profile Pack, 2 edn*, Macmillan Magazines: London

Paniagua H (1995). The Scope of Advanced Practice: action potential for practice nurses, *Br J Nurs*, **4** (5)

Pilkington Hudson (1980). In: *OXFAM, Pass the Port Again*, Christian Brann, Cirencester: pp111

Royal College of Nursing (1990). *Professional Portfolio*, Scutari Publications, Harrow

Steinaker, N W and Bell M R (1979). The Experiential Taxonomy, Academic Press, New York

UKCC (1990). *Post Registration and Practice, Project Discussion Paper*, UKCC: London

UKCC (1990). *The Report of the Post Registration Education and Practice Project*, UKCC: London

UKCC (1992). *The Scope of Professional Practice*, UKCC: London

UKCC (1994a). T*he Future of Professional Practice—the Council's Standards for Education and Practice following Registration*, UKCC: London

UKCC (1994b). *Register*, UKCC: London

UKCC (1994c). *Registrar's Letter 20/1994*, UKCC: London

UKCC (1995). *PREP & YOU*, UKCC: London

UKCC (1995b). *Registrar's Letter 3/1995 25 January*, UKCC: London

Welsh National Board (1991), *Professional Profile*, London: Austen Cornish Publishers

Index

Advanced practice 58
Advanced Practitioner   42
APEL   8, 52, 69, 70, 71, 72
APL 12, 32, 70, 71, 72
Assessment of Prior Experiential
Learning   68
Assessment of prior learning   64
   experiential   64

BJN portfolio pack   77

Career development   7
CATS   6, 8, 32, 47, 61, 62, 64, 72
Clinical supervision   42
CNAA 62
Contracts for high-quality care   55
CREDIT ACCUMULATION   62
Credit Accumulation and Transfer
System 61
CREDIT EXEMPTION 62
CREDIT TRANSFER   62
Curriculum Vitae   13, 16
CV   17, 18, 22, 33

education   4, 6, 23, 26
   development 6
   evidence of   23
   General 23
   Higher   24, 32
   informal   26
   professional   24
ENB Framework   44, 47
ENB Framework   42

ENB Higher Award   72
ENB Personal Portfolio pack 63
ENB Professional Portfolio   48, 73
ENB Professional Portfolio
folder   68

Five day of study   36

General Practice Nursing   50
Goal
   categories 35
   setting   34
Goal setting   33
goals
   Personal   33
   professional   33

Higher Award   6, 12, 17, 42, 47, 54,
58, 63
   requirements for   48

Learning outcomes   68

Midirs (Midwives Information and
Resource Service) Midwifery Po   78

Non-nursing employment 29
   Previous   29
Notification of Practice 38
nurses
   Opportunities for second-level   54
   second-level 54
Nursing

Community Children's 50
Community Mental Handicap50
Community Mental Health50
District 50
General Practice 50
Occupational Health 50
Public Health 50
School 52
nursing employment
    Previous 29
Nursing Times Profile Pack 76

Open University 24

periodic registration 33
Personal development 7
personal portfolio 2, 4, 10, 42
personal portfolio or profile 1
personal portfolios and profiles 2
Personal Professional Profile 39
Personal profiles 5
PIN 22
preceptor 40
    role of 41
preceptor 58
Professional practice 58
profile packages 73
profiles 33, 42

Project 2000 24, 54
Provider 56
Purchaser 56

Return to Practice 43
    programme 43
Royal College of Nursing
Professional Portfolio 79

Specialist practice 49, 58
    definition 50
Specialist Practitioner 42
Stages in making a claim 65
support
    provision of 40

UKCC profile requirements 43
UKCC requirements 36
UKCC Specialist Practitioner 72

voluntary work 30

Welsh National Board Professional Profile 78